Praise for *Mad Sisters*

"Without sugar-coating, Susan Grundy recounts the emotional roller-coaster of caring for her older sister after the teen is diagnosed with schizophrenia. Beautifully written, *Mad Sisters* breaks your heart only to lift it moments later, as Grundy's actions reveal the havoc caused by a serious mental disorder, the horrific toll it takes and a sister's unyielding and abiding love. An indispensable book for those of us who love someone with a mental illness."
—Pete Earley, *New York Times* best-selling author of
Crazy: A Father's Search Through America's Mental Health Madness,
a finalist for the Pulitzer Prize

"*Mad Sisters* is a raw and honest memoir that bravely confronts and unpacks complex family dynamics, traumatic experiences, and the unbreakable bond between siblings. It's an emotional rollercoaster of a read, and well worth the ride."
— Mark Henick, Principal & CEO of Mark Henick Mental Health Media,
author of *So-Called Normal: A Memoir of Family, Depression and Resilience*

"With Mad Sisters, Susan Grundy gives a moving testimony to love, sisterhood, and stick-to-it-iveness, conveying her sister Nancy's lifelong struggles—including an endless stream of hospitalizations and psych drugs, and all their many harms—with a raw, insightful honesty that brings both of them vividly to life. Their relationship is complex, and their story isn't easy, but the bond between them is tangible and inspiring. The result is a powerful ode to human resilience."
—Amy Biancolli, author and former family editor for Mad in America,
whose mission is to serve as a catalyst for rethinking psychiatric care

"Susan Grundy's older sister saved her from drowning in childhood, forging an unbreakable bond between them. Now, as they navigate middle age, Susan feels an unyielding duty to reciprocate. With their parents unable or unavailable to support a daughter with chronic mental illness, Susan takes on the mantle of Nancy's protector and advocate. She battles a mental health system fraught with gaps and ineffective, sometimes dangerous, treatments. She struggles with personal questions that haunt her day and night: Where do her responsibilities begin and end? Is she fostering dependence or nurturing the independence they both crave?

"This poignant, finely drawn narrative alternates between vivid childhood memories and the sisters' tumultuous adult lives. The author captures the full spectrum of their emotions: jealousy and gratitude, grief and joy, exasperation and acceptance, resentment and reconciliation. Se̶ ̶i̶n̶ ̶l̶ insurmountable di-

T0273929

lemmas dissolve into laughter under Susan's relentless prodding and Nancy's sharp wit. By the book's end, you'll want to envelop them both in a heartfelt embrace. Susan Grundy's memoir is an important contribution to awareness and understanding of the impact of chronic mental illness on siblings."

—Deborah Kasdan, author of *Roll Back the World: A Sister's Memoir*, one of the 100 Best Indie Books of 2023—*Kirkus Reviews*

"An insightful account of the challenges faced when caring for a sibling with a mental health condition."

—Michael Shann, Carers UK

"In the gripping and heart-wrenching memoir, *Mad Sisters* author Susan Grundy weaves a powerful story of two sisters bound by love, torn by despair and obligation, and tested by the unyielding hardships of mental illness. I laughed. I cried. Sisters Nancy and Susan are inseparable, their bond a forcefield of hope through the blackest times. Laced with humour and a dogged need to stay connected as sisters, the book delves deep into the near-impossible daily struggles family members face, revealing the devastating lifetime impact of Nancy's condition on all their lives.

"With raw honesty, Susan Grundy exposes the gaping holes in the medical system and the often catastrophic imperfections of medications that promise stability but deliver inconsistency. Their journey is one of resilience, navigating a labyrinth of hope and hopelessness, understanding and misunderstanding. *Mad Sisters* is a poignant exploration of the human spirit, an unflinching look at the realities of mental illness, and a powerful reminder of the enduring strength of sisterhood. This compelling narrative will leave readers reflecting on the importance of compassion, and the need for systemic change."

—Susan Doherty, author of the award-winning *The Ghost Garden* and *Monday Rent Boy*

"Susan Grundy's tender memoir tells of her decades-long struggle to love and care for her older sister Nancy, diagnosed with schizophrenia at age thirteen, who can be in turn infuriating, heartbreaking and endearing. Full of stories told with empathy both for Nancy and for herself, this is a family saga you won't want to put down."

—Vikki Stark, author of *My Sister, My Self: The Surprising Ways that Being an Older, Younger, Middle or Twin Shaped Your Life*

"I finished reading Susan Grundy's memoir with tears in my eyes. Lifelong responsibilities to support her ill sister—mostly as her primary caregiver—have not compromised her unswerving commitment and unabated compassion, despite sometimes feeling frustration, resentment, and sometimes hate. Mental illness can be difficult to forgive when behaviour towards your closest caregivers becomes inexcusably harsh; yet she remains her sister's mainstay through stormy and turbulent times. Susan's memoir, oscillating between past and present, opens a window into a life marked by the pain and travails evoked by mental illness. . . . Being a young carer without recognizing it, Susan was subjected to the inevitable impact of mental illness that ravaged her sister's life starting at thirteen. Taking on her sister's physical ailments as if they were her own and bearing the associated stresses, Susan became her ultimate protector, accepting her lot with uncanny generosity.

"While Susan does not often lash out at the health care system, there is an implicit message that needs to be heard: mental illness is a 'family affair'; an imperfect, fragmented health care system victimizes not only the diagnosed member but their entire entourage."

—Ella Amir, Executive Director, AMI-Québec, Allies in Mental Health

MAD SISTERS

Susan Grundy

Memoir

RONSDALE PRESS

MAD SISTERS
Copyright © 2024 Susan Grundy

All rights reserved, including those for text and data mining, A.I. training, and similar technologies. No part of this publication may be reproduced, stored in a retrieval system, or transmitted, in any form or by any means, without prior written permission of the publisher, or, in Canada, in the case of photocopying or other reprographic copying, a licence from Access Copyright (the Canadian Copyright Licensing Agency).

RONSDALE PRESS
125A – 1030 Denman Street, Vancouver, B.C. Canada V6G 2M6
www.ronsdalepress.com

Book Design: David Lester
Cover Design: Dorian Danielsen
Cover Artwork: Nancy May Grundy

Ronsdale Press wishes to thank the following for their support of its publishing program: the Canada Council for the Arts, the Government of Canada, the British Columbia Arts Council, and the Province of British Columbia through the British Columbia Book Publishing Tax Credit program.

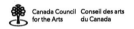

Library and Archives Canada Cataloguing in Publication

Title: Mad sisters / Susan Grundy.
Names: Grundy, Susan (Susan Frances), author.
Identifiers: Canadiana (print) 20240401158 | Canadiana (ebook) 20240401174 |
    ISBN 9781553807186 (softcover) | ISBN 9781553807193 (EPUB)
Subjects: LCSH: Grundy, Susan (Susan Frances)—Family. | LCSH:
    Caregivers—Canada—Biography. | LCSH:
    Caregivers—Family relationships—Canada. | LCSH:
    Schizophrenics—Care—Canada. | LCSH:
    Schizophrenics—Family relationships—Canada. | LCSH: Sisters—Canada—
    Biography. | LCGFT: Autobiographies.
Classification: LCC RC514 .G78 2024 | DDC 616.89/80092—dc23

At Ronsdale Press we are committed to protecting the environment. To this end we are working with Canopy and printers to phase out our use of paper produced from ancient forests. This book is one step towards that goal.

Printed in Canada

To my beautiful and darling sister

1

MY SISTER SAVED ME FROM DROWNING when I was five. It was a sticky July afternoon, the peak of summer in Ontario's Muskoka Lakes region. Nancy was at the opposite end of the pool, in the deep end. Three years older, she could do things I couldn't, swimming being one of them. Our parents were nowhere in sight, engaged in one of their adult activities at the resort. They'd left me in my sister's charge following their truncated tennis match two days earlier when I'd chased a stray ball and had run into the net cable. I still have a dent where the wire sliced my nose.

The pool was a choppy sea of bouncing children. I gripped the rough cement and edged closer to my sister, who was looking in my direction from the deep end. She didn't wave back. Water covered my shoulders, my neck and then my chin. Standing on tiptoe, I reached for the floating line of red and blue flags. A tidal wave from a human cannonball ripped my other hand from the edge and my toes could no longer touch bottom. I flapped my arms and screamed, but the cry was drowned out by squealing children. My sister's face flashed before me. She had moved closer to the red and blue floating flags and was treading water effortlessly, the usual blank expression on her face. Didn't she see that I was in trouble? My heart sank with the possibility that she mistook my wild thrashing for swimming. I swallowed more water and slipped below the surface.

Someone grabbed my armpits, pulled me back to the shallow end and nudged me up the steps. Cold, damp fingers steered my wobbly body towards a grassy area next to the pool, where I collapsed face down on a towel. My ears were buzzing; I couldn't understand what the person leaning over me was saying. I pushed up to my knees and swayed for a second or two, then folded forward into a crouch, resting my forehead on the towel that reeked of Coppertone lotion, a fake flowery smell I'd never cared for. Without warning, my stomach started to pump. I raised my head seconds before the resort's all-you-can-eat buffet breakfast gushed out of my mouth. A second eruption followed, then another. Emptied, I rolled onto the grass, away from the stinky mess. My sister was standing over me, motionless and silent, her face a dark outline against the blue sky.

I assumed a cross-legged position, wiped the spit off my chin and adjusted the bathing suit strap that had slipped down my right arm. She sat beside me, legs bent to one side in her girlish style, and stared at the pool full of bouncing children, a slight frown on her face, perhaps because of her vomit-soaked towel.

I jabbed her with my elbow.

"How come you didn't help me sooner?"

"I saved you, didn't I?" Her voice was low, monotone.

I poked her again, harder.

"You took your time. Mom and Dad told you to watch over me."

She rubbed her side, the one that I had poked.

"Mom and Dad told you to stay in the shallow end," she retorted.

I was too weak to argue. My throat was burning from puke and pool water. The sun was beaming, but I was sitting next to a block of ice. I hugged my shoulders and squeezed myself into a ball. In the end, neither one of us would tell our parents about the near drowning, a rare act of complicity.

In July 2019, on a similar sticky summer afternoon, I sat in a hard vinyl chair next to my sister in Dr. Byrne's waiting room at the External Clinic for Psychotic Disorders, a white-walled space with a forty-inch television and a window looking onto the sprawling grounds of Montreal's Douglas Hospital. Nancy had first met Dr. Byrne in the 1980s, during her extended stay on Perry 2C, a locked ward that has since been shut down. A budding psychiatric doctor at the time, he was now in his early sixties like us.

The man across from us in the clinic was slumped over in his chair, possibly asleep. His clothes reeked of nicotine. Thankfully, Nancy had quit smoking, a rare feat for someone with a schizoaffective disorder. A testament to her determination.

"Do I know you?" Nancy asked the slumped-over man.

A long time ago, my sister was reserved. Now she spoke to everyone. The man lifted his head in slow motion. His mouth was open, and a bit of drool had escaped onto his unshaven chin. He was younger than I had expected, a baby face with cloudy blue eyes. He stared at me as if I'd asked my sister's question. I scrolled through my phone, in no mood to converse with strangers, mentally ill or otherwise. An old email from a friend caught my attention, an invitation that had never been answered. I started to type. *Sorry for not answering sooner . . .* then stopped, distracted by Nancy's fingers tapping against the arm of the chair. Her uncontrolled shaking was from years of taking lithium, a distressing side effect of a drug meant to stabilize mood.

"That gadget's more important than me," she growled loud enough for the receptionist behind the glass window to hear.

I saved the email along with the other unfinished emails and turned to her.

"I'm trying to catch up with my life and work. Not easy to do with all the phone calls and problems you want me to fix."

"What problems?"

"How about the ones from yesterday? The window latch, the television. There was a third one . . . I can't remember what it was now."

"Darling, if you don't remember, then you didn't take care of it."

I dropped the phone into my bag.

"Let's not argue, okay? I'm still recovering from your blast on the sidewalk. Go home to your sucker husband. Real nice, Nance."

"You hung up on me last night."

"Do you remember why?" I asked.

"You had better things to do than talk with your sick sister."

"I hung up because you were disrespectful."

"That's ridiculous. You're the one who was disrespectful."

The man across from us was no longer slumped over. We had his full attention, the sister sideshow being more interesting than the swirling lines on the clinic's linoleum floor.

"Keep your voice down," I whispered.

Nancy stood with great effort, weighed down by medication and bitterness. She accidentally knocked over one of her dollar store shopping bags. A spiral notebook slid onto the linoleum.

"Did you write another poem?" I asked.

Nancy often picked up the pen following our arguments, her way of having the last word. Her poems were riddled with clever rhymes and innuendos only a sister would understand. Unfortunately, the prose was transient. She'd rip out the page and throw it away, as she did many things. Understandable, her brain was cluttered enough.

The notebook was pressed against her chest. She was glaring at me.

"These are my notes for Dr. Byrne. Private notes."

I had no interest in her written complaints that she would read and rip out, then crumple in a fist and cast into Dr. Byrne's garbage can with surprising aim. I had my own grievances. My presence at the clinic usually signalled a problem, and today was no exception. But before speaking up, I would have to wait for her to finish talking. After all, she was the patient, not me.

Shopping bags in hand, Nancy shuffled towards a mother and twenty-something daughter sitting at the end of our row. The women looked like twin sculptures, one thirty years older than the other. They had the same high cheekbones, aquiline noses and shoulder-length dark, wavy hair. The mother, younger than us, wore a sleeveless white blouse and floral-print skirt—grown-up clothes compared to my rainbow-patterned hippie sundress and Nancy's turquoise T-shirt and black leggings. The mother's eyes were fixed on the view through the window, the century-old maples dotting the verdant grounds of the Douglas Hospital, formerly the Protestant Hospital for the Insane. An unopened paperback rested on her lap. The daughter's dark, flashing eyes were checking out my sister from head to toe.

"I've seen you around," she said to Nancy. Her voice sounded rough, hard.

Nancy lowered the bags to the floor and slapped her thigh.

"I knew there was someone I would know in this room!"

Not a surprise, Montreal is a small community for English speakers, even smaller for those with psychotic disorders.

"I think we met at the Wellington Centre," Nancy said.

"Maybe."

The daughter studied Nancy's turquoise T-shirt and then pointed down the row at me.

"Is that your sister?" she asked.

Nancy smiled. "She sure is. Susie Q. Two husbands, two children, two homes."

I winced.

"She's the older sister?"

"No!" Nancy and I cried in unison.

The mother turned from the window and smiled at me, an empathetic gesture from one caregiver to another. The half-moon shadows under her dark eyes reminded me how tired I was, barely recuperated from the battles with my sister the afternoon and evening before. Another argument would surely erupt, not in Dr. Byrne's office where we practiced self-control, but in the restaurant during lunch, in the car on the way home or in the course of our multiple daily phone calls that carved a huge chunk out of my life—time I could use to write, answer emails, visit my two adult children, hang with friends, help my husband at the cottage or simply stare into space. Had this worn-out mother sitting a few seats down from me figured out, as I had, that setting boundaries with a mentally ill loved one doesn't work? Or maybe her daughter was easier to deal with than my sister, required less attention, had fewer demands. From the mom's lined face and the daughter's hard voice, I had my doubts. When a family member falls sick, everyone succumbs, at least those who stick around.

Dr. Byrne appeared in a tweed jacket, grey flannels and woven tie. Nancy commented on how smartly he was dressed. She was highly skilled at handing out compliments, often directing them at strangers, her way perhaps to connect with the world. The doctor smiled and signalled to the mother and daughter. Our turn was next, according to Nancy, who had returned to her seat beside me. The slumped-over man, meanwhile, had vanished. I welcomed the peace and quiet in the waiting room, no one left to talk to.

"Look at that, Sue." Nancy pointed at the swim competition on the television screen.

I yawned. "Swimming has always been your thing, not mine."

"I could have been in the Olympics."

"Darling, you're still a good swimmer. I don't understand why you don't take advantage of the Benny pool. It's a minute walk from your place."

"My dear little sister, don't tell me what to do."

"Yes, dear."

I was wasting my breath. Again.

She nudged me, a sharp little dig. "Remember how I pulled you out of the pool? You were drowning!"

My nose burned from the memory of chlorine. I pictured my sister watching from the deep end just before my head had sunk below the surface. A minute longer and I would have drowned. Back then, did she feel like I felt waiting to see Dr. Byrne, trapped by responsibility? Is that why she had hesitated to save me? Or was the pause just my imagination?

Nancy hobbled off to the bathroom with great purpose, her crooked walk reminiscent of a wounded warrior. My sister had saved me once. I'd saved her a hundred times since. Was I beholden to her forever? Sitting in the External Clinic for Psychotic Disorders on that sticky July afternoon, I had no hope that my life would ever change.

2

WHEN MY SISTER AND I WERE TEN AND SEVEN, I almost drowned a second time halfway through another family holiday. We were following the footpath next to the river in Richmond-upon-Thames, ten miles southwest of Waterloo Station, in Central London, and two hundred miles southeast of my father's birthplace in Manchester. I would appreciate these facts only later in life. Back then, the distances were useless numbers our mother had asked us to memorize, numbers my sister rattled off with no effort. It was the summer of 1964. "I Want to Hold Your Hand" held the number one position on the *Billboard* pop singles chart. I thought the song was ridiculous. Holding my father's hand had prevented me from running ahead on the footpath to chase after the mother duck and her cute babies, likely the most exciting event that would happen that afternoon. Protesting was pointless; I was a prisoner in my father's iron grip. My pleas to join my sister in the kayak had also been denied. I wasn't a strong enough swimmer. I wasn't even allowed to help guide the kayak with the rope my father held in his other hand. My mother was no help. We'd left her on a park bench with her tourist guidebook, looking for more facts to teach my sister and me or, worse, choosing another boring old church to visit. I didn't understand the fascination with churches. It wasn't like we ever went to them back home. I looked up at the cloudy sky and prayed for rain.

The clouds parted and the July sun bounced off the river. My sister's strawberry-blond hair was showered in sparkling light, a halo. Wrapped in a bulky life jacket, she held her back perfectly straight in a posture I could never maintain—and still can't.

"Lower the paddle a little deeper in the water and pull towards you," said my father.

She followed the instructions. The front of the kayak carved a perfect V in the water.

"Well done. Carry on!"

My father picked up the pace, dragging me alongside.

"Nancy gets to do everything."

Normally, I would be scolded for whining. Thankfully, my father wasn't listening. He was staring ahead, eyebrows furrowed as they often were, likely thinking about his work even though we were on vacation. I looked over my shoulder. My mother on the park bench was no longer visible. I was alone in my misery.

Without warning, the kayak veered away from us. The rope jerked, and my father tripped on something, a tree root maybe. His grip on my hand tightened as he pitched towards the riverbank, still holding onto the rope, determined to not let go of either daughter. My fingers were released only when we hit the river, narrowly missing the kayak. I entered the Thames headfirst. The water was thicker than a pool or a lake. I couldn't see past my flailing hands. The muddy liquid sucked me into spinning circles. I couldn't tell which end was up. My feet touched something slimy and solid, the river bottom maybe, and I pushed away with all my strength, holding my breath even though my chest was close to bursting.

A pair of strong hands scooped me out of the water and lifted me into the air. I blinked at a moustached man in a black suit with round silver buttons down the front. The shiny badge on his helmet was inches away, so tempting to touch. It was the first time I had seen an English policeman up close. I smiled even though my heart was pounding and my clothes were a muddy mess. I wanted to show him that I was brave.

"You're okay, luv," said the policeman, lowering me with care to the grass beside where my mother was standing, the tourist book tucked under her arm. He turned and offered a hand to my father, who was clinging to the edge of the embankment. Like many English people of his generation, Dad had never learned to swim.

"I arrived just in time," said my mother.

"Did you see what happened?" I asked, rushing my words. My heart was still racing.

"I see you need swimming lessons as soon as we get home," she replied in her schoolteacher voice.

Lessons during school summer holiday were undeserved punishment. I scowled at the kayak. My sister was holding the paddle like an expert.

"Can I take lessons too?" she asked, even though she already knew how to swim.

My mother nodded and turned to my father.

"You should sign up as well, Norman," she said in the soft tone reserved for him.

"Good idea, Lorna," replied Norman.

A monster-sized black cabby carried us to our hotel in Central London. On the way, my sister pointed out Big Ben, Parliament and various bridges. How did she know all these things? Why did she care? I was more concerned about the clothes that stuck to me like a second skin and the large imprint my river-soaked bottom was making on the leather seat. My father paid our driver with soggy paper bills from his wallet. One by one, we pushed through the hotel's revolving door. To my horror, the lobby was humming with guests. Four o'clock—we'd arrived in time for tea. My soaked sneakers squeaked across the marble floor, drowning out the delicate clinking of cups on saucers. Heads turned. Murmured comments. My cheeks burned with humiliation as I followed my family into a crowded elevator. I scuttled to the back corner, crossed my arms and glowered at the red velvet–panelled wall.

"What floor would you like?" Nancy asked a tall woman in a short dress. Her white leather boots looked brand new.

"Sixth, please," the woman replied. "How sweet. Are you in charge?"

Nancy blushed. "Only of my little sister," she replied.

The tall woman turned and stared down at me. Her fake lashes looked like spider legs.

"You're soaking wet!" she cried.

"So is my dad."

She glanced over at my father. For some reason, he didn't look nearly as wet.

"What happened?" she asked.

"I fell in the river."

"Off a boat?"

"I wasn't allowed in a boat. A rope pulled me in."

I had hoped she would ask more questions. Maybe she would pity me. But she had already turned back to my sister.

"You know, you look just like the actress Hayley Mills."

"*The Parent Trap* is my favourite movie," Nancy said, beaming.

I'd heard about my sister and Hayley Mills too many times. No one ever compared me to a famous person. The elevator door opened on the fifth floor. I rushed out. It was pointless to run down the hall, however. Nancy had the key to our room. She was in charge.

Nancy escorted me to the bathroom and poured a hot bath as per our mother's instructions. I wasn't fond of bathing, but showers were much worse. In a bath, at least my face stayed relatively dry, even when I leaned back to wet my hair. In a shower, water bullets filled my eyes, ears and nose making it impossible to see, hear or breathe. I waited for my sister to leave before stepping into the tub. Our parents' voices on the other side of the wall were muffled. Ice clinked in a glass. Drinks before dinner meant we would be eating late again, not that my sister ever complained. I scrubbed the funky smell of the River Thames from my arms and legs and then pulled the plug. No need to linger. The job was done. The dirty ring around the bathtub was final proof.

I slipped into the hotel bathrobe five sizes too big and pirouetted in front of the bedroom mirror, flapping the sleeves like white wings. A book on London hid my sister's face. I was wasting my time. She wouldn't find me funny. Instead, she would tell me to pick up my wet clothes and scrub the tub. She was not my friend. I kicked at the carpet, slumped down on my side of the bed and reviewed the afternoon. My father was wrong; I would have been safer in the kayak. My mother had sided with him, as usual. It was my sister's fault the rope had jerked from our dad's hand. She hadn't offered me an apology. Nobody had. An ice cream with sparkles would have been nice, or a bag of chocolate kisses from the hotel gift shop. I would even have accepted a boring tea biscuit from the hotel lobby. Two near-drowning incidents: it was clear my family was unreliable. I pulled the duvet over my head and made a vow to escape.

Dr. Byrne appeared again. This time he beckoned us to follow. Our turn. Before standing from her seat in the waiting room, Nancy redistributed the contents of her dollar store bags with a logic that made no sense to me. The shuffling of the wallet, notebook, glass case, Kleenex and list of prescription medications was her anxious way of taking inventory. Towards the end of his life, our father had performed a similar ritual, convinced he'd lost something when he hadn't. Sometimes I catch myself doing the same thing. An orderly disorder.

With her dollar store bags intact, Nancy exited the waiting room in the direction of Dr. Byrne's office. She moved at full steam despite her crooked walk. I followed at a safe distance.

"You're still on that thing?" Nancy asked from the office doorway. She pointed at the phone in my hand.

"Just turning the ringer off."

"Wish I had a phone that I could turn on and off."

I rolled my eyes. "You always tell me you don't want one. Your fingers shake too much."

"Maybe I want one now."

"I'll be happy to buy you one."

"I can buy it myself, darling. I know what I want. A flip phone."

"Darling, you'll need my credit card."

"I'll use my debit card."

"You need a credit card to set up the account. Like we do with everything else. The pharmacy, the dentist—"

Nancy threw her arms in the air. "You win, darling sister!"

A credit rating was on the list of things my sister would never have. She was a dependent, unable to earn her living. I lowered my voice. "It's not a contest, Nancy. I'm just trying to help."

"It would be more helpful to not look at your phone."

She turned from me, champion of the last word.

Dr. Byrne stood at attention beside his desk, feet together, arms by his side. I wondered how much he'd heard and if he felt my pain, not that it made any difference. Her doctor, not mine. He was highly respectful of my sister and allowed her to speak freely without interruption, his way of diagnosing her emotional condition, I suspected. A patient man with many patients—over eight hundred, we were once told.

"Where do you want me to sit?" I asked my sister.

She studied the two worn wooden visitor chairs and pointed to the one closest to the door.

"That one."

The three of us settled. Dr. Byrne opened a file.

"How is everything?" he asked my sister.

Nancy cleared her throat. "Actually, I would prefer the chair Sue is in."

I rolled my eyes a second time, picked up my tote bag and changed places. Nancy remained standing, holding her imaginary power.

"Did you have a good vacation, Dr. Byrne?" she asked, rocking back and forth without moving her feet.

"Yes, thank you. The week went by very quickly."

"A week? My sister and her husband go to Costa Rica for months!"

My fists clenched. The hit was small, but it stung regardless, like the fire ants under the palms in our tropical garden. I missed Casa Verano and the jungle beside our house, the creepy-crawly things less so.

"Used to go," I said in a quiet voice. "We recently sold the property and bought a cottage in the Eastern Townships. Colder, but much closer, a ninety-minute drive."

"Yes, Nancy told me," Dr. Byrne said. His tone was bright, cheerful.

Nancy grunted. "I've only been invited once this summer."

Dr. Byrne flipped through the file.

"Everything seems fine. Your blood levels are all within normal range. How are you feeling?"

She raised her hands. "The lithium is too strong. See the shaking?"

"I do," he said and made a note in the file.

Nancy opened her notebook.

"I have a few other problems I wish to discuss."

Dr. Byrne lowered his pen and leaned back in his chair to listen. I braced myself for the onslaught. My sister unfolded the medication schedule the pharmacist had provided with her weekly Dispill, a blister pack that organized her medicines into separate compartments for different times of the day for each day of the week. The lengthy list of drugs made me cringe, a reminder of how lucky I was. Lithium, Clozaril, Latuda, Seroquel, Klonopin, et cetera, et cetera. She waved the paper in the air.

"I have no clue what some of these pills are for, but they all make me constipated. I blocked the toilet three times in the past two weeks. My stools are hard like stone, and when I block the toilet, I have to wait around for the plumber because there's no janitor in my building. Susie fixed the toilet once with her plunger. She also changed a light bulb on my kitchen ceiling. But she's busy with lots of important things to do. Don't get me wrong. I'm grateful to be living in a decent condo, so much better than a group home or the hospital. But there are problems. My new knee is still not working properly. I'm not swimming, which is too bad because it's good for my knee. My sister had a pool in Costa Rica, and now she swims at a lovely lake near her cottage whenever she likes. As I said before, I've only been invited once this summer . . ."

As Nancy spoke, the oversized watch on her wrist tapped against Dr. Byrne's wooden desk at a pace that reminded me of our father's clicking metronome in the days when he practiced the allegro passages from Schubert's "Sonata No. 14" in A minor. I sank deeper into the visitor chair, my head throbbing from the urgent items that needed to be discussed. Would my sister tell Dr. Byrne about her increasing reliance on me, the multiple phone calls, the constant complaints and demands? More likely she would tell him what happened yesterday, how I had screamed at her outside the café. It was the only way I could be heard above her roar.

Despite the vow declared over half a century ago, I had not escaped from my birth family, at least not from my sister. I was stuck to her like glue. Krazy Glue. The more I tried to push away, the tighter the strands of sister DNA pulled us together. A barely audible squeak escaped from my throat. Dr. Byrne glanced in my direction. Had he heard my pathetic plea for help? He turned back to Nancy. After all, she was the patient, not me.

3

IN THE EARLY 1960S, THE TORONTO URBAN SPRAWL had not yet reached the field behind our split-level bungalow in Etobicoke or the little woods at the end of our block. My first memory is being tied to the garden tap at the side of the house, a creative measure taken to prevent me from wandering beyond the backyard, where I would hide in the tall grass. That afternoon, my mother was hanging laundry on the clothesline with Nancy's help. Neither paid attention to my cries. The rope was generous in length; I could almost reach the white, shaggy dog similarly tied in the yard next door. Somehow, I wiggled free, proof to my young self that persistence pays off. Rather than risk being caught, I ran in the opposite direction from the clothesline and the field, not stopping until I reached the middle of Tettenhall Road, where I lay straight as a pencil. At the age of three, I was not only adventurous, I was also invincible; a car could easily pass over or around me. The stunt was a stupid one, I realized when five minutes passed without any traffic. I returned to the garden tap and waited, untied, for my mother to finish hanging the laundry. She stopped using the rope after that.

Our father's middle-management position at British American Oil required frequent travel, especially following the takeover by Gulf Oil Corporation. Our brilliant and bored mother was left stranded in Toronto suburbia, residing within a twenty-five-kilometre zone of where her mother, grandmother and four other generations were buried. Fuelled by amphetamines prescribed for weight loss and Sweet Caporals that she smoked from a black cigarette holder, she poured her ambition into managing the household. An executive secretary before marriage, she banged out our weekly chores on an Underwood typewriter and posted lists on the kitchen wall, a practice that would persist into our late adolescence. Meals were prepared with minimum fuss: beef, pork and lamb roasts with canned peas and potatoes. When our father was out of town, we ate Swanson TV dinners directly from the aluminum foil trays that were later tossed into the garbage. No plates to wash! My favourite TV dinner was the fried chicken with mashed potatoes and stewed apples. Our mother preferred anything to cooking, even ironing. She had been born in the wrong era and, given a choice, would never have had children—her words, not mine. Luckily, her eldest daughter was eager to step up. Nancy craved responsibility. I was too young to understand that what she really wanted from our parents was approval and love. I'd already given up on the former.

Watching over her wandering little sister was not an easy assign-ment, even though Nancy knew all my escape routes, including the gap between our father's prized rose bushes that led to a nice lady's house with an endless supply of Girl Guide cookies. The neighbourhood kids, closer in age to Nancy, were of no interest to me, especially the bully who punched me in the lower back for tagging along. During those preschool years, the local dogs and cats were my best allies.

My freedom to wander was compromised with the advent of kinder-garten, although I was grateful to make friends my own age. By the time I entered grade 3, I had wiggled out of the sister-chaperoned walks to and from school. As a result, the boundaries of my solo explorations expanded exponentially. Eight years old, I discovered the little woods at the end of our block. My secret forest was a magical place. In its centre, hidden from the street, stood a tall conifer with a pointy top and wide-reaching branches covered in long needles and scaly cones—a perfect climbing tree. The smell reminded me of Christmas candy canes and sugar plum fairies.

It had been a bad day. The substitute teacher in my grade 3 class had accused me of being a "furniture mover" because I kept shifting my chair. She forced me to stay after school even though it was the second to last Friday before the summer holidays. My eyes burned. I'd done nothing wrong, no clue that the strawberry Jell-O powder my mother had given me for recess had made my sugar level surge. I only knew that the snack made me the envy of the other kids.

After detention, I ran the four blocks to my secret forest, climbed onto a stump and grabbed hold of an overhanging limb on the climbing tree. I walked my feet up the trunk and hung upside down by my knees. I paused there for a brief topsy-turvy swing, then hoisted myself up and started the ascent. Several branches higher—it might have been two, but it felt like ten—I opened my knapsack and pulled out a half-eaten peanut butter sandwich left over from breakfast, one of five sandwiches I'd been instructed by our mother to make and put in the freezer on Sunday night. "It saves time on school mornings," she had said. I tossed the sandwich to the ground and peeled open a chocolate bar. A breeze picked up, making the leaves in the surrounding trees applaud. The memory of the undeserved detention faded. I imagined a time before split bungalows and sprawling backyards when Etobicoke was called something else. My grade 3 teacher had written the word in large chalk letters on the blackboard. ABODIGOK. It means where the alders grow, she had said. I peered down from my branch, wishing for someone from Abodigok to appear.

"Come down right now, Susie, or you're in big trouble."

My sister was standing directly underneath, hands on hips. My sister-boss. The disapproving look on her face reminded me of my Friday afternoon piano lesson due to begin in five minutes.

"In a sec." Pointless to rush, I was already late, already in trouble.

"How come you didn't eat breakfast?" she said, waving the half-eaten peanut butter sandwich she had picked up from the ground.

"Wasn't hungry," I replied.

"Where'd you get that chocolate bar?"

Like a parent, she had X-ray eyes.

"Did you buy it with loose change from Dad's dresser?" she asked, sounding a bit like the grade 3 substitute teacher.

I took a bite and started chewing, assessing my options. I could remain in the climbing tree like the time I locked myself in the bathroom when I refused to eat fish soup. Nancy had eaten every drop. What kind of kid likes fish soup?

"You going to tell on me?"

We both knew she would. I made my way down, pausing on each branch to take another bite of the chocolate bar, in no rush to face the consequences. I'd grown too old for bum spankings. My father would likely use the bristle side of the hairbrush on my arm. Maybe I'd be given a small portion for dessert, or worse, no dessert at all. I lagged ten feet behind my sister all the way home and held my breath when I walked through the front door. But fate played in my favour; the piano teacher was running late! I used the bonus time to practice my scales. At the end of the lesson, she stuck a gold star on my music book. Our father, recently returned from Pittsburgh, was in a rare jolly mood at dinner. Nobody mentioned the chocolate bar. My mother passed me a generous portion of cake, which I gobbled down and then, as always, waited for Nancy to finish hers, as per the table rules. With great precision, she scooped up a small bit of the delicious dessert and slowly raised the spoon to her mouth. I suspected she was trying to torture me, her way of holding sister power.

During the Etobicoke years, our parents would sometimes take us downtown to Lichee Garden on Elizabeth Street, one of the first Chinese restaurants in Toronto to serve liquor, a phenomenon my parents raved about for reasons I didn't understand at the time. They sipped on martinis while my sister and I speared maraschino cherries in our Shirley Temples. Nancy refused to duel with the miniature paper umbrellas; the childish behaviour was beneath her. Instead, she listened to the grown-up conversation. Our father sounded miserable when he spoke about the office. Why he worked at such a horrible place was beyond me. Nancy nursed her Shirley Temple while I stuffed sugar cubes into my pockets.

After dinner, our father steered the white Plymouth Valiant onto the Gardiner Expressway. Lake Ontario was hidden in darkness on our left. On our right, the Royal York Hotel gleamed, a castle made of golden bricks. My belly was full of egg rolls and pineapple chicken. It was a struggle to keep my eyelids open.

"Can you keep a secret?" my sister whispered in my ear.

"Huh?" I rubbed my eyes.

"You were adopted."

She slid back to her side and stared at the road ahead, no further discussion. I studied her upturned nose, the way she clasped her hands together in her lap, her freshly shampooed, neatly combed strawberry-blond hair, the even fringe of bangs across her forehead, the way she didn't move like she was made of stone. My hair was a mop of blond curls, a bird's nest, according to our mother. I was unable to keep my hands or any part of me clean or still for very long. I fantasized about my real sister, the one from whom I was separated at birth, just like in the movie *The Parent Trap*. She was just like me.

The next morning, I pulled the family album from the living room bookshelf.

"Who's that in your belly?" I asked my mother and pointed to a photo of her in a black maternity dress pushing Nancy in a baby swing.

"You, of course."

"Are you sure?"

"Don't be silly. Look at the date on the photo. August 23, 1957. A week before you were born."

Not convinced, I flipped through the rest of the album.

"How come you don't have more pictures of me when I was a baby? You have lots of Nancy."

"You kept us busy."

"Didn't Nancy keep you busy?"

"She was quiet. No trouble. Not at all like you!"

I didn't tell my mother that my sister had told a lie. My mother would have never believed me. Nor would she understand how I had secretly wished the lie to be true. I left my mother and the photos, slinked up the stairs to my room and wiggled under the bed to retrieve a candy bar purchased with more loose change taken from my father's dresser. The chocolate would have tasted even sweeter if I could have shared it with a sister. But I was an only child; at least that's how it felt.

Dr. Byrne pushed up from his desk, a signal that the appointment had come to an end. We'd run out of time, and I hadn't had a chance to voice my urgent concerns. At least the shaking had been addressed.

"Thank you," I said in a small voice.

I rose from my chair and Dr. Byrne moved to the doorway. Nancy remained seated, fussing with where to file her new prescription with the reduced lithium dosage. So many choices with her complex bag system. She tucked the paper inside one of her small zippered pouches and then stuffed the pouch inside a larger one. And still, she was not done. I shook the doctor's hand and made a beeline for the hallway and the glass doors. Nancy would catch up. She was never far behind.

I waited on the sidewalk a half-block from the clinic, hoping Nancy would remember where I parked and wishing she would hurry up. The heat was making my sundress stick to my skin in an unpleasant way. A colony of gulls flew over boulevard LaSalle and landed on the narrow

18

stretch of grass next to the river. The rapids glinted with sunlight. The air would be cooler by the water. I tried to remember: in all the years I'd driven down to the Douglas Hospital, had I ever indulged in a river walk?

"Yoo-hoo, Sue!"

Nancy was approaching, walking with the mother and daughter we'd met in the waiting room. She was laughing, relieved after all the unloading in Dr. Byrne's office. I turned away in a lousy mood.

"You'll never believe this, darling," Nancy said. "These lovely ladies live two blocks from my place!"

I smiled politely and prayed that the mom and daughter didn't need a lift. They didn't. They were parked directly in front of me. The daughter disappeared inside their car. The mother hesitated on the sidewalk. Her dark eyes shifted from me to Nancy, then back to me.

"You know," she said. "Out here in the bright light, you two look even more alike."

I laughed, a fake little "Ha ha," and wondered what the woman saw. Nancy and I had nothing in common—inside or out.

Nancy tapped the back of the car. "Can you open the trunk?"

"Why bother? Just leave your shopping bags on the passenger seat floor."

"There's no room for my feet."

Nancy gets what Nancy wants; convincing her otherwise is a waste of time.

I slipped into the driver's seat, popped open the trunk and scowled. The cumulative impact of demands now made her most minor request extremely irritating.

"I can't close the trunk," she called out.

"Press the button, darling."

"Which button?"

"The one with the picture of an open trunk."

"I don't see a picture."

Nancy's resistance to new technology was frustrating. Was this a rebellion or a sign of cognitive decline from her illness, like the way she no longer had the focus to read a book cover to cover? I preferred the former theory; the latter one was too sad. In my haste to exit the car, my elbow knocked over a bottle, pouring water over the driver's seat.

"Fuck!"

I slammed the door shut.

"Did you just swear at me?" she asked.

My sister's voice was charged, ready for a fight. I didn't bother to explain that I was swearing at the spilt water and not at her. She wouldn't believe me. And maybe she would be right. We stood our ground, two feet between us. She raised her palms towards me like a shield. I wavered, aware of a passing pedestrian. Nancy lowered her arms. The storm between us passed. My cheeks felt strangely warm. I wondered if they were as flushed as my sister's. I pushed the button and the trunk lowered.

Nancy whistled by breathing in, her special way.

"Fancy car, this Audi. Must have been expensive."

"I got a deal, remember? The car was two years old."

"Remember how Dad and Mom paid for the last one?"

"They didn't pay for all of it. And besides, Dad and Mom are dead."

It sounded mean, what I had said, but I hated the way she talked about our parents like they still played a role in our lives. So what if they had given me some money for a car? Did she remember how I used to drive our parents to Beaver Lake every week, how I chauffeured them to all their doctor appointments, how I did the same for her? She didn't care about such facts. I had a car and she didn't.

"Get in, Nancy. Let's go."

She handed me an envelope.

"What's this?"

"For your birthday."

"My birthday is five weeks away!"

"Open it."

The envelope was decorated with swirls of blue and pink chalk pastel. A folded page was tucked inside, next to a greeting card that had been deliberately left blank for repurposing. My sister had inherited our parents' spendthrift gene. The compulsion to acknowledge birthdays weeks in advance was part of her restless pattern. I dropped the card in my bag and unfolded the paper, a page torn from her agenda. The painting was simple, minimalist compared to the complex abstract art she produced in her student years. At the top, she had drawn a couple of upside-down balloons with their strings floating up towards the sky. At the bottom was a sketch of the Audi, the four wheels not connected to the car. In the driver's seat sat a stick figure with an arm out the window, waving.

Happy Birthday! Incredible! What dynamite! It's Susie Q, that's right. Rolls with the punches. Puts up a fight! She looks like 21. All right!

The poem, like others she had written about her little sister, made me uncomfortable and slightly suspicious. I was rarely a recipient of Nancy's free-flowing compliments. Rolling from punches and putting up a fight did not feel very flattering. The message was upside down like the two floating balloons she had drawn. Regardless, I would stash the poem with the other cards in one of the drawers in our father's campaign desk or in the filing cabinet where I kept her tax returns, insurance policies, lease renewals and utility bills. My sister was free of such tedium and responsibility. She didn't require a desk or a place to file papers. I suspected she didn't keep the cards I gave her longer than a day or two, same for her drawings. The exceptions to her throw-away rule were the colourful scarves and table linens she created on a loom at L'Atelier, a non-profit studio promoting art for mental health. Their supportive and structured approach pushed her to persevere. She was fiercely proud of her stunning woven art and with good reason.

"Thank you for the poem, my dear." I returned the torn-out page to the envelope.

"Where's the birthday card?" Her voice was a little sharp.

"In my tote bag somewhere."

"Take it out before it gets crushed."

Her eyes watched closely, pulling me back in time. Nancy was always the meticulous child. Susie was the messy one.

"I'm starving," Nancy said. "Let's go to a restaurant."

"I would rather drop you off at your place if that's okay."

She looked at me with puppy dog eyes. "Darling, I have nothing in the fridge."

She won. How could I say no?

"Okay. Let's go."

I pursed my lips and turned the ignition. Ideally, I would have driven Nancy directly home as planned. But our world was far from ideal.

4

I SAT ON THE EDGE OF THE BED in our split-level bungalow on Tettenhall Road and refused to budge. My mother ignored me. Preoccupied by preparations for our upcoming move, she instructed my sister to pack up my room. Nancy had emptied hers hours earlier. One by one, my treasures were removed from the shelves, the dresser and the little desk. My sister wrapped each item in newspaper with a focused precision that annoyed me.

My nine-year-old feet kicked the bed frame.

"I don't wanna leave Etobicoke," I muttered, loud enough for my sister to hear.

"We have to leave. Dad has a new job."

Her words were drab and dull like the December sky outside the window. I wanted to leap off the bed and shake her awake. Who cares about a new job? Did she not realize we were leaving our home, never to return, never mind that it was the week before Christmas? Two men in dark blue coveralls appeared in the doorway. I slid off the bed and flattened myself against the wall while they stripped the rest of the room bare. The empty space looked very small.

Our Plymouth Valiant followed the bright orange Allied Van Lines truck down Tettenhall Road. I whispered goodbye to our split bungalow, to the sweet old ladies and their cookies, to my elementary school four blocks away where my grade 4 friends were at their desks. Nancy hadn't said a word about having to leave her new junior high school where she had started grade 7. We turned the corner and picked up speed. My secret forest flashed by, no time for a wave. I wanted to tell my father to slow down or, better yet, turn the car around. I looked over at my sister. They might listen to her if she would only speak up. She was staring out the window at the blur of passing bungalows. I slumped into my seat, defeated.

The storm started just past Kingston and turned into a blizzard at the Ontario-Quebec border. Our car was immersed in a white cloud, the windshield wipers flapping at full speed. Our father had told us that Montreal would have more snow than Toronto and that there was a park a block from our new home in Westmount with a steep hill for sliding. We could learn how to ski. Admittedly, the idea excited me. Where we had lived in Etobicoke, the land was completely flat. He had also told us about Expo 67, which was starting in the spring. He called it a world's fair. The snow was more appealing.

"Can we unpack the toboggan when we get there?" I asked from the back seat.

My mother turned and frowned. "Your father needs to focus on the road."

I didn't understand what was so difficult about driving. The car was barely moving. All he had to do was follow the blinking red tail lights of the car ahead.

I poked the back of my mother's seat with my toes.

"How much longer?" I whispered.

"Stop kicking," she replied, this time not turning.

"How much longer?" I asked again.

"Settle down, Susan." Our father's Manchester accent was more pronounced when he was provoked. In those early years, I assumed everyone from England sounded like that.

Nancy's eyelids were closed. A map of Montreal open on her lap. I had no idea what she found so interesting about a bunch of criss-crossing lines and street names. No wonder she'd dozed off. I stretched one leg across the back seat.

"You're on my side of the seat," she said in a quiet voice my parents couldn't hear.

I surveyed her with suspicion. She sounded too awake to have just woken up. I snuggled into my corner and started to count the swishes of the windshield wipers. At the speed we were driving, surely, I would reach one million.

When my eyes opened, the snow had stopped falling. We were parked in front of a two-storey square house made of dull red brick, very ordinary. No sign of a garage, the front yard was puny, not enough room to throw a Frisbee. At least our new home was an impressive size, with an entranceway on each side.

"Which one's the front door?" I asked.

"On the right," replied my mother.

"What about the one on the left?"

"That's our neighbour's house. It's semi-detached."

Semi-detached meant nothing to me. All I knew was that we were moving into half a house. Something lodged in my throat. I couldn't speak. I stepped out of the car, my legs feeling shaky. All the houses on the block were made of the same dull red brick; all the front yards were puny. My sister appeared beside me. I grabbed her arm.

"Moving was a big mistake," I whispered.

She opened her mouth, but no words came out. Her lips came together in a small frown. The silence gave me hope. Maybe for once, she would agree with me. The air running in and out of her nostrils made a small wheezing sound like when she had asthma. Her eyes were fixed on our new old-looking home with a boring flat roof, nothing like the modern split-level bungalow we'd left behind.

"Do you feel as bad as I do?" I asked.

She shuffled from one foot to the other.

"Do you?" I asked again.

Nancy looked at me with our father's steel-blue eyes. "Come on. We have to help." She stepped away, my hold on her arm broken. She didn't fool me. For sure she was feeling bad. What kid wouldn't under these circumstances? My fear of the future turned into anger with the present. My sister had betrayed me again. With little choice, I followed her inside.

My mother promised that the crack running across my bedroom wall would be repaired. "It's the original plaster," she said. I didn't care about plaster. I cared about the wall collapsing. I slumped down on my bed, the plastic wrap still on the mattress, and stared out the window at my view of a neighbour's red brick wall. The room smelled like old lady perfume. I could hear boxes being ripped open and paper rustling in my sister's room, the one with sunlight, and a balcony. I walked over to my box of treasures and began pulling them out, one by one.

The Quebec school system was very different from what my sister and I were used to, like so many other aspects of our new home. The curriculum was almost a year ahead of Ontario's. Thankfully, our report cards from Etobicoke were good enough (especially Nancy's) that we were spared being pulled back a grade. Quebec had no junior or middle schools like the one where Nancy had started in Etobicoke; Quebec high school began at grade 7 and ended at grade 11. Our move to Quebec coincided with a new education act that created the two-year CEGEP (Collège d'enseignement général et profesessionnel) program. Before the act, students entered Quebec universities directly from high school. No wonder the curriculum was ahead.

The playground at Roslyn Elementary was made of asphalt and bordered by a chain fence, a prison compared to the grassy field behind my school back in Etobicoke. At Roslyn, girls and boys used separate entrances, which made me wonder if Westmount boys were bullies. My new grade 4 classmates had been together since September, many of them since kindergarten. They could speak French and had already been taught how to divide. Kids asked me questions no one had asked before. What did my father do? Did we have a country house? Was I Protestant? Jewish? (My mother had to tell me what Jewish meant.) The cliques were impenetrable. I was referred to as "the new girl from Toronto" until the morning we lined up at the nurse's office for the oral polio vaccine. The cherry-flavoured syrup was sickly sweet, and I struggled to keep it down. My status quickly changed to "the new girl from Toronto who puked all over her French book."

Nancy never told our parents about her first day at Westmount High School, how she had taken the wrong bus, ended up lost downtown, and circled the block for an hour before she found a policeman. She arrived at the classroom flushed and flustered, her armpits dripping in sweat. Thirty pairs of eyes stared her down, "the new girl from Toronto." Her hands still shake when she talks about it. That first winter in our new home, Nancy was invisible to me, shut off in her bedroom to catch up with the Quebec curriculum. Her persistence paid off. By the end of the school year, she was one of the top students in her class and had forged a few friendships with similar-minded students.

My parents were pleased with Nancy's diligence. They had no clue what was really going on. Years later, Nancy described the mounting pressure that had fuelled her long study hours and how she'd sometimes blanked out during the day, exhausted from the strange ideas that haunted her at night. She held onto her thoughts like dark secrets. Our parents mistook her silence for good behaviour. After all, she had always been the quiet child compared to her chaotic little sister. They had no idea of the powerful emotions taking hold during that first year in our new home—pathos, envy, guilt and extreme frustration—and that she was slowly disconnecting from family, from everything.

Late morning, I shuffled into the kitchen on the last Saturday in June marking our second Fête St-Jean-Baptiste holiday weekend in Montreal. Etobicoke was a year and a half in the past. I had graduated from grade 5, only one year remaining at Roslyn Elementary. Nancy had finished grade 8, her second year at Westmount High, with honours. She was seated at the kitchen counter facing the window, her back to me. Her spoon clanged against the cereal bowl filled with our parents' bland bran buds. I rubbed the sleep from my eyes, opened the cupboard and reached for the Honey Nut Cheerios. Our parents were talking in the living room, positioned at their usual "recliner chair" stations.

"Lots of girls want short hair these days," I heard my mother say.

Since I could remember, my mother had insisted that short hair was practical for my unruly curls, especially since I didn't fuss about my appearance. But at ten years old, I no longer appreciated being mistaken for a boy.

"I'm sick of short hair!" I shouted.

"They're not talking about you," Nancy said. I swivelled towards the cool voice and the cereal box slipped from my hands. The hair that once fell to the middle of my sister's back had been cut in a perfectly straight line just below the ears, exposing a beauty mark on her pale neck.

My mother stormed into the kitchen and I pointed at the back of my sister's head. Nancy turned to face us. She was a different person, older. She looked like Twiggy, the pretty model on the magazine cover. Nobody would ever mistake her for a boy, even with cropped hair. But something didn't add up. Her hair had been long when I went to bed.

"But . . ."

"She did it herself," my mother said quickly, cutting me off. "And a fine job, too."

Her voice was strained, like she'd been smoking more.

"When?"

"Four-thirty this morning."

My mother's matter-of-fact voice was confusing. Who cuts their own hair in the middle of the night? I shook my head.

"That's nuts."

"She had insomnia."

Ten years of my mother's rough voice had taught me to drop the subject. I scanned the kitchen for more clues. The sewing scissors were lying to the left of the kitchen sink next to a clear plastic bag full of my sister's dead hair. Repulsed and slightly queasy, I returned the box of Honey Nut Cheerios to the cupboard. I'd never heard of insomnia before. Hopefully, it wasn't contagious.

The Fête St-Jean had been hit by a heat wave. We lay low that afternoon. The evening provided little relief. I gulped glasses of lemonade in front of a boring movie while my parents sipped gin on the back porch. Nancy's door was closed; she'd gone to bed early. Nothing to do, I did the same. The nighthawks were restless that night. They seemed to have picked our roof to circle over, calling out their sad cry. I tossed and turned in bed. My darling sister had given me her insomnia bug.

Something woke me when it was still dark, muffled voices from my sister's room. I threw off the sheet and listened. Was that laughter or crying? Strange that my door was closed; I always kept it open. I tiptoed out of my room and into the hallway. My parents were leaning over my sister's bed, illuminated by the small reading lamp on her desk. The balcony door and window were wide open and the curtains drawn apart. Still, the air was thick. Dead air, with an acrid sickly scent. A cool gust on my back gave me shivers. My parents had left their air-conditioned bedroom door open, something they never did.

"Go back to bed, Susan." My father waved his hand without looking up.

I ignored his order, unable to take my eyes off my sister. Her eyes were half-open, the lids fluttering like butterflies. Words came out of her mouth jumbled together in a strange language that made my stomach gurgle. My mother leaned over the bed and pinned my sister's flailing arms. I clenched my hands into fists and took another step forward, driven by morbid curiosity.

"Wake up, Nancy," my father said in his sternest voice, the intimidating Manchester accent.

My hands relaxed. She was having an awake-nightmare, like when I saw a line of creatures across my windowsill, their skinny legs dangling like Muppets. A high fever, my mother had said. I looked over at my sister's windowsill. No Muppets there, only her cactus plant next to the alarm clock: three o'clock in the morning.

My mother rushed past me and returned seconds later with a damp washcloth. She dabbed my sister's forehead. Nancy shot up to sitting. Her eyes were balls of fire. She screamed, a piercing shriek that brought my hands to my ears and glued my feet to the floor. My mother's worried face turned ghostly white and my father's hands were shaking. The scene of frightened parents was far worse than any nightmare. The air became even thicker and I started to cough. My father's go-to-your-room glare unglued my feet. I shuffled backwards to my bed and pulled the sheet over my head, leaving a little hole for air as if I were a whale—a nocturnal ritual that I've since kept all these years. The thin cotton shield stuck to my damp cheeks and forehead. I squeezed my eyelids together. An explosion of blues and purples replaced the image of my parents leaning over my sister's bed. I pictured the nighthawks circling over our house. Their sad cries were even louder than the screaming from my sister's room. I squeezed my eyes tighter. Giant birds' wings etched the blue and purple background with black Vs. For years afterwards, I dreaded nightfall when the nighthawks congregated. Their cries triggered dread, a dead weight in my chest. I never told my parents; they had enough worries.

I woke to daylight with a metallic taste in my mouth from a bitten lip. My teeth were sore and I had a small headache. My room was intact: a half-eaten apple on the bedside table, dirty clothes heaped on the floor, treasures lined up on the shelves. Our neighbour was mowing in their backyard, and the poodle on the other side of our back fence was yapping as usual. I tried to recall the horror scene in my sister's room and the strange things she had said, the jumble of words, names of people she claimed to be—Cleopatra, Rudolf Nureyev among them. She had asked if she was Hitler because, if so, she needed to throw herself from the balcony. Or did I remember correctly? Details started to fade. I rolled out of bed and opened my door that someone had closed. Nancy's room was empty. Her sheets and blanket had been removed from the mattress. I ventured down the hall in search of my parents, my arms tightly crossed against my chest. I felt numb, like I was filled with nothing, stunned.

I kept my promise and stopped at a restaurant in Verdun on the way home from the appointment with Dr. Byrne. Nancy ordered a club sandwich. I drank coffee. Afterwards, she asked me to drop her off at Pharmaprix, which was a convenient half-block from her one-bedroom rental condo on avenue Benny; she had a new prescription to fill. Alone at last, I sped west along Sherbrooke ouest, a seven-minute drive to my home at the bottom of the hill in Lower Westmount. My second husband, Keith, had just arrived from our cottage in the Eastern Townships, his base since retirement. He tolerated my need to spend time in the city—even if I didn't do much apart from visit my sister and write. Over dinner, Keith listened to my rant about Nancy, what she had said in Dr. Byrne's office and what I hadn't had a chance to say. The topic of my sister dominated the conversation in our marriage more than I cared to admit. Lately, the compulsion was out of control.

Keith went to bed early, perhaps exhausted from my monologue. I joined him at midnight, still wired. The events of the day repeated in my head. My sister's remark about how she had been invited only once to our cottage still irked me. Did Dr. Byrne realize how exhausting Nancy's behaviour was when she stayed overnight? She treated Keith and me like servants from morning to night, delivering one command after another to satisfy her needs. Nancy needed to be the constant centre of attention. When criticized or slightly corrected, she would launch into a jealous rage. Keith and my two adult children, Sarah and Willy, walked on eggshells around Nancy. Lately, my steps had become heavy. Crunch. Crunch. My patience was drying up. These thoughts and others played havoc in my head while Keith slept beside me. I tried listening to his gentle inhales and exhales. Sometimes that helped put me to sleep. But I was too wired. That bloody coffee at the restaurant in Verdun! If I had gone straight home, I would have made myself a calming chamomile tea. I sighed and pulled at the sheet, a little too roughly. Keith stirred but, thankfully, didn't wake.

Maybe I was making too big a deal about this. My poor sister had been given a lousy deal, after all. Her life had been ripped from her at age thirteen. She was right about my two homes, two kids, two husbands, the Audi—I was privileged, the lucky one. A second invitation to the cottage before the end of summer was a small thing to ask. She could come for her birthday, maybe stay two nights. I yawned. Finally, sleep was coming.

In my dream, I was standing on the deck of a large vessel, more like a freighter than a passenger ship, surrounded by wooden crates. Someone behind me yelled, "Take cover!" The air suddenly thickened and the sky grew dark. An evil force was invading the ship. I imagined grotesque Frankenstein monsters staggering like zombies, their inhuman arms stretched forward to grab their victims' necks. I took shelter inside one of the wooden crates, but the top cover wouldn't close properly. I climbed out of the crate and crept along the deck towards the bow of the ship. A lifeboat was waiting in the choppy water below, an opportunity for escape. I took a step towards the top rung of the ladder. My sister called out behind me. She was begging me to stay. My feet wouldn't move; they were glued to the deck. I woke up gasping and threw the blanket off my head. I'd forgotten to make a proper air hole to breathe.

5

THE SIGN ABOVE THE COUNTER at the nursing station read *Psychiatric Ward*.

"The floor is off-limits to young visitors," the nurse said to my parents.

I pushed up on my toes. "I'm turning eleven in two months!"

The nurse leaned forward and patted my head, like I was a dog.

"Sorry, sweetie, you need to be sixteen."

My heels lowered in defeat. Nancy was so close, down the hall in one of the rooms; my cheeks burned from the injustice. Walking between my parents, I kicked at the black specks on the linoleum floor on our way back to the fifth-floor elevators. I knew better than to make a fuss. This wasn't their fault.

My parents parked me on a bench in Cabot Square, which faced the Montreal Children's Hospital. I was given strict instructions to stay put until they returned from their visit with Nancy. I nodded with enthusiasm, eager to check out the new toys I'd chosen at the hospital gift store. I bounced the little red ball and picked up one jack. On my second bounce, I picked up two. Cheating a little, I dropped the jacks close together and picked up five. Satisfied, I opened the box of miniature puppets. They magically came to life on my fingers. Each one took a turn starring in my plays. After a few minutes, I returned them to the cardboard box, wished them pleasant dreams and replaced the lid. An older couple walked by and smiled. I looked beyond them, at the hospital, and counted the floors until I reached the fifth, then swivelled on the bench to face the recently renovated Montreal Forum. Through the enormous glass window, two gigantic escalators crossed like hockey sticks. Maple Leaf Gardens didn't have anything as fancy. My allegiance started to shift that sunny summer afternoon as I stood next to the bench in Cabot Square in awe of the cars racing down Ste-Catherine ouest and the throngs of people on the sidewalk. Suburban Etobicoke suddenly looked a little dull.

"Schizophrenia is like a cork popping from a bottle," I told solicitous adults over the next few weeks, repeating what I had overheard. My hands were folded in my lap and my legs were crossed, just how my sister would have sat. The adults showered me with compliments. They told me I was handling it well. I didn't feel like I was handling anything. The doctors would fix my sister and send her home. I was more worried about my distraught mother and her muffled crying from the other side of the bedroom door.

My prediction turned out to be incorrect. The doctors at the Montreal Children's Hospital couldn't fix my sister. Following a delay caused by a hospital-wide hepatitis outbreak, Nancy was transferred to the Allan Memorial Institute, an intimidating white stone mansion perched on the edge of Mount Royal. "The Allan" was about to make headlines with breaking news of LSD experiments conducted on patients under the authorization of the Central Intelligence Agency. Nancy had narrowly missed that fate. Under the care of Dr. Unwin, she was discharged near the end of August, just after her fourteenth birthday.

A few days after her discharge, I stood in the doorway of her bedroom. An imposter sat on the edge of my sister's bed and stared out the balcony window. Her shoulders slumped forward and her head was bowed, chin against chest like a string puppet at rest. I knocked on the open door, unsure how to approach.

"Lunch is ready."

I'd done my best to sound cheerful, like everything was normal. But normally, my sister would be calling me for lunch and not the other way around.

The imposter sister turned her head in slow motion. Her eyes were glazed, mouth slightly open. I couldn't help but stare.

"Coming," she said, dropping the consonants. My mother had explained how the medication slowed down Nancy's muscles, including the tongue.

"You okay?" I asked, scanning her face, looking for clues of the old Nancy in this new empty shell.

She lifted herself from the bed with great effort. Her sweater had ridden up, revealing her belly.

"Coming," she repeated.

We sat in our usual places at the mahogany dining room table, parents at each end and sisters across from each other. Nancy raised a spoon to her lips. Vegetable soup dripped down her blouse. Our parents ignored the mishap and kept chatting. For once, they didn't talk about problems at the office. They were discussing plans for the afternoon. Their eyes kept coming back to my sister.

"You've developed quite an appetite, luv," said our father, eyeing Nancy's empty soup bowl.

"It feels good." Her voice was small, diminished.

"Want mine?" I asked.

Our father pointed at my bowl. "Finish it, Susan."

I made a face and reached for the bread. Our mother refilled her wine glass and turned to our father.

"Norman, let's go out for a walk after lunch. Such a beautiful day. We could have tea in the garden afterwards. What do you think, darling?"

"Excellent idea, Lorna," our father replied. "A stroll would do us good."

Bad idea, I thought. Our father's "strolls" were marathons, lasting two to three hours, fun for grown-ups and deadly dull for kids. I hoped my sister's condition would cut the stroll down to an hour. We left the dirty dishes in the sink, a phenomenon that had never happened before, and the four of us stepped out the front door. The photo our father took on the porch that afternoon is one of the last to appear in the family album. Our mother is wearing a tweed suit and cat-eye sunglasses, the same pair I now own. Her short hair is tinted silver, making her look much older than forty-five. She is flirting with the photographer, as she did for most photographs. One leg is posed in front of the other, her skirt raised six inches above the knee. I'm squatting on the top step in jeans and a sweatshirt, a bored smirk across my face. My hair still cropped short, I could be mistaken for a boy. Nancy stands behind me, holding our mother's hand. Her legs are awkwardly apart, covered by a knit skirt and knee-high socks. Her hair has grown an inch since she cut it off at the end of June. Her face is pasty white, the corners of her mouth lifted in a small, sad smile, and her gaze downward, away from the camera. She looks fragile, like fine porcelain. In her hand is a turned maple leaf, one I'd picked off the lawn and handed to her. Though it was late August, fall had arrived early that year. In the black and white photo, the leaf is a dark grey.

We descended the hill towards the end of our block, Nancy still holding our mother's hand. The turtle pace was pure torture. Our father called me back when I raced ahead.

"We have to take it slow," he whispered.

Rakes paused as we passed the dull red brick homes on either side of our street. The perfect weekend weather had brought everyone outdoors. Some neighbours waved, some said hello, some were silent. Everyone watched. The word on the street was out. The girl from Toronto had been discharged from the psych ward. I stepped off the sidewalk, away from my family, and kicked through the leaves that had been swept onto the road, my chin held high to show the neighbours I wasn't the crazy one.

We stopped at the lookout in Murray Hill Park, at the top of what would become a toboggan run in the winter, something to look forward to. Our mother pointed out the church steeples in Lower Westmount and the water beyond.

"The Saint Lawrence River," Nancy said, sounding almost like her old self.

Our parents looked at each other and smiled. I smiled too. The family stroll was not such a bad idea after all. Nancy was talking, and her cheeks had become flushed. She looked less broken. Our father snapped another photo and suggested we press on. Nancy turned from the lookout and tripped. She landed in a heap on the cement path.

"You're bleeding," I said and pointed at her knee. It was a bad scrape.

She didn't check her injury. Instead, she stared up at the sky in a way that made me shiver. Despite what it had seemed moments earlier, the stroll had failed to snap her out of the stupor. Our parents helped her to stand and we headed home for tea.

I sat cross-legged on our back lawn and bit into the shortbread my aunt had shipped from England the summer before. It tasted like buttered cardboard. Nancy's hands hung motionless down the sides of the wicker chair. I stretched my legs and poked her foot with mine like I used to do in the back seat of the car. She didn't budge. I poked harder, a jab like one I would administer under the dining room table. The fingers on her right hand twitched and her head turned in my direction. She stared, without blinking, at my outstretched foot. I retracted my legs and hugged my knees into my chest. I wanted to run away, but there was nowhere to go.

From time to time, Nancy has shared snippets of her hospitalization at The Allan. The memories are blurred by time and medication, but the stories are genuine; they belong to her. Thirteen years old, she was the only adolescent on the ward. Pumped with tranquilizers, she joined the group therapy sessions with patients closer to our parents' age. Many of them were male. Some made sexual innuendos that made her skin crawl. Occasionally, she was allowed outside on the hospital grounds. Nobody warned her that the drugs would make her skin sensitive to the sun. An afternoon outing on the grounds ended with a wicked burn on her arms, neck and face. She stepped into the shower to relieve the pain and mistakenly turned on the hot water instead of the cold. Her screaming brought staff running. They wrapped her in bandages and locked her door. On August 10, 1968, she spent her fourteenth birthday looking out a dirty window at the passing cars on avenue des Pins. From that summer forward, she would be reeled in by psychiatrists, nurses, therapists, our parents, group homes and in the years to come, her little sister. She would never experience the gift of independence that begins with adolescence.

Our mother offered me another piece of shortbread. I shook my head; my half-eaten cookie had been tossed into the peony bush when no one was looking. I pulled out a fistful of grass from the lawn and blew the blades out of my hand.

"Did you make a wish?" our mother asked.

I smiled and nodded, knowing she made wishes too. Two weeks earlier, before my sister's discharge, our father had led my mother and me on a stroll to Westmount Summit. When the rain had started to fall, we took cover in nearby St. Joseph's Oratory. The basilica was packed with devout worshippers. We settled in the back row, my parents on either side of me. Three drowned rats. I looked up, way up. Our father had once told us that the dome was as high as St. Paul's in London. An organist, hidden from view, was playing from an upper gallery.

"Bach," our father said. His eyes were closed.

Our mother leaned forward and dropped her knees onto what I had mistaken for a footrest. Her arms lifted and her palms came together, all ten fingers pointing at the dome, the heavens. Her lips opened and closed without making a sound. I stared, my own mouth agape. I'd never seen her pray before. Our father, lost in Bach, didn't notice. It occurred to me, as it did again sitting on the grass in our backyard, that there was little difference between a prayer and a wish.

The neighbour's grey tabby squeezed through a gap between the wooden fence posts. It settled on the grass next to my sister's wicker chair. Under different circumstances, I would have leaned over and grabbed the cat I'd been chasing all summer. Instead, my eyes were on my sister. Her arm had unfrozen and she was petting the cat with slow and deliberate strokes. Don't give up hope, I wanted to say to our parents. But I was only a kid, so I didn't. The only thing I could do was to try to make them happy.

A few weeks had passed since our appointment with Dr. Byrne and my sister's shaking had not improved; in fact, she was worse. Nancy agreed that I should request another lithium reduction. I left a message with the clinic and climbed the stairs to the second floor, morning coffee in one hand, phone in the other. The home office was waiting, the day cleared for writing, not that my day needed clearing. I no longer required an agenda since I'd neatly filed my marketing business in the hall closet four years earlier. Appointments were now scribbled on bits of paper. My social circle had eroded in the years following the end of my first marriage. Friendships made in Costa Rica had washed in and washed out like the tide. The new cottage was perched on the side of a mountain with a breathtaking view of the northern end of the Appalachian Trail—lots of deer and no people. My nest in Montreal was also empty: Sarah had moved to Toronto; Willy lived in nearby Saint-Henri and worked long hours. Nancy remained the person I saw most often. Apart from visits with Keith at the cottage, somehow I'd become like my parents: a hermit.

My desk was orderly: writing pad and pen on the right, laptop dead centre. I sipped more coffee and checked my phone to make sure the ringer was turned on. Nancy had promised to call right after her annual scan. Yesterday I reminded her, as I did every year, that the endocrine tumour the surgeon had removed from her pancreas ten years earlier was rare and the likelihood of another was low. The doctor had cut out her spleen as well—apparently, she didn't need one. I massaged a cramp below my rib cage. My sister's physical ailments often felt like mine.

The pancreatic tumour wasn't her only brush with cancer. Nancy had stage zero leukemia. The hematologist assured us the asymptom-atic condition was stable and had nothing to do with her medication. I was skeptical. Clozaril played havoc with white blood cells and was prescribed only when other antipsychotic medications failed. Nancy also had developed type 2 diabetes, a common condition for someone struggling with a psychotic disorder. What's next, I wondered? The life expectancy associated with schizoaffective bipolar disorder was ten to fifteen years less than the general population. My sister was sixty-five; I didn't want to do the math.

I pushed up from my desk and climbed into the hammock chair Keith had attached to the beam in my office ceiling, my hanging refuge. The swaying calmed me. For a few seconds, the blur of greenery out the bay window transported me to the stone patio at Casa Verano, where I would nap in the same swinging chair every afternoon. The phone rang and I lowered my foot to the floor.

"Can you help me, darling?" asked my sister.

The cramp below my ribs returned.

"Is everything okay? What happened with the scan?"

She paused. I held my breath.

"Oh, that," she replied. "I'm fine. I need you to call the landlord. I have a problem and I'm in a rush to get to L'Atelier to finish a throw blanket."

Relief flushed through me like a toilet draining. My sister was okay. I half-listened to the problem, a closet door that wouldn't slide. I prom-ised to call the landlord and we hung up. I returned to my desk, know-ing I should deal with the faulty closet sooner rather than later because she would be calling back many times to check. The cramping was re-placed by a burning sensation in my stomach. I was no scientist, but the tumour, leukemia and diabetes were likely linked to the psychotropic drugs my sister had taken for most of her adolescent and adult life, drugs that didn't keep her mentally stable, drugs that didn't make her happy. Prescribing was trial and error. Even the doctors had told me so. Would she have been better off taking nothing?

6

SEPTEMBER 1968, THE DAY BEFORE I would start grade 6, creaking floor-boards on the staircase woke me at two o'clock in the morning, followed by the click of the kitchen light switch and the rattling of the cutlery drawer, the one that always got stuck. My hearing is above average; back then, it was razor-sharp. I wiggled towards the edge of the bed, the side closest to the open door. The freezer opened and closed with a small thud and a kitchen stool scraped across the linoleum. Then silence. I fell back to sleep.

Seven hours later, my parents were sipping coffee in the living room and the kitchen was empty, my sister nowhere to be seen. The dirty spoon in the sink reminded me of my interrupted sleep. I opened the freezer, found the evidence and marched into the living room waving a near-empty carton of ice cream.

"Look at this!" I cried.

My mother's face appeared from behind the Sunday *New York Times*. Her right eyebrow arched in a frown. "Norman, I bought that ice cream yesterday," she said.

My father lowered his newspaper and scowled. "Slovenly!"

He had called me that name many times. This was a first for my sister. In the two weeks following the hospital discharge, a new personality had emerged from the empty shell of my zombie sister, one that made me a little less hopeful that the old Nancy would ever wake up. The new sister was disruptive and unpredictable. Her unruly outbursts and irrational accusations crossed the boundary of teenage tantrums. She spent most of the day in bed and raided the fridge at night. At my suggestion, my mother stashed our Hershey chocolate bars in the wooden slot on the underside of the dining room table. Secret hiding places were my specialty. Other strategies were less effective, like the way my parents tried to shout out my sister's unruly behaviour. I observed the screaming battles from doorways. With the adult disapproval no longer directed at me, I had become the good daughter.

My parents folded their newspapers and stood up from their recliners, synchronized. I followed them upstairs, the ice cream carton still in my hand. Nancy was lying on her back under the sheets, arms and legs stretched out in a four-pointed star. Her mouth was half open and she was snoring, a high-pitched whistle. Her eyes popped open when the drapes parted with a furious yank, flooding the bedroom with light. She clutched the top of the sheet. Her gaze shifted from our mother to our father to me, reminiscent of Dorothy in *The Wizard of Oz* with Auntie Em, Uncle Henry and the three farmhands gathered around her bed. "There's no place like home," Dorothy says before the movie credits start to roll. The scene in my sister's room would not end like that.

Nancy glared at the piece of evidence dangling from my hand.

"Snitch," she muttered.

I slipped into the hall, safe from the line of fire, close enough to watch.

"Did you go down to the kitchen in the middle of the night?" my father asked in his clipped English accent.

"Maybe."

"Maybe? What kind of an answer is that?"

"I guess I did."

"What did Lorna and I tell you about stuffing yourself? It's piggish."

"Maybe I'm a pig."

My mother ripped the sheet off my sister.

"It's not healthy to stay in bed this late," she shouted.

"I don't want to get up."

Rage etched a trail of blotchy red lines across my father's face. Don't ever be fooled by the reserve of an Englishman. I took a step back.

"Listen to your mother. GET UP!"

"GET UP!" Lorna repeated. She stood next to my father at the foot of the bed, her arm wrapped around his elbow to pull him closer. The familiar image of my parents united in fury and taking turns yelling made me uneasy, even if I was invisible, even if their rage was no longer directed at me. I retreated down the hall with my hands cupped over my ears. Being a snitch wasn't as much fun as I'd thought. In fact, the ordeal had me a little queasy for some reason. For the first time since we'd moved from Etobicoke, I looked forward to the new school year. Anything to get out of the house.

The next morning, I waited outside the girl's entrance in the lineup for Mr. Bowker's grade 6 class. I still hadn't found a permanent friend since we'd moved to Westmount, apart from Alana, and that hadn't worked out so well. Our sleepover at her cottage had ended abruptly when I was overwhelmed by homesickness; Alana's mom had to drive me home. Shame and confusion still haunted me. I surveyed the line-ups in the schoolyard, wondering whom I could play with at recess, if anyone.

The girl ahead of me had long wavy hair that smelled of Herbal Essences shampoo. She was no more than an inch taller than me. We would likely be the shortest in the class. *Beth* was stitched in pink wavy letters across the back of her denim knapsack. She turned around and smiled with large shiny brown eyes that reminded me of a puppy. Her face was pale and perfectly round, like an angel.

I looked down at the ground, trying to think of something clever to say.

"We have the same shoes. Did you get them at Tony's?"

"Naw," she said. "That store's too expensive. We bought these in the States and smuggled them across the border."

I was intrigued. Smugglers!

The bell rang and the line moved forward. We marched past the nurse's room, where I had ingested that dreadful cherry vaccine a year and a half earlier, and past the principal and vice-principal standing at attention in front of the office door. Beth grabbed my hand when we reached the classroom and pulled me to a desk beside her, two rows from the front.

"We'll be close to the action," she whispered. "Mr. Bowker stands on his desk when he's upset. That's why they call him Mr. Barker." She opened her pencil case and passed me a chestnut, perfectly round like her eyes.

"Wow. Where'd you find this?" I hadn't seen such a perfect chestnut since Etobicoke.

"Villa Maria."

I had ridden past Villa Maria on my bike plenty of times but never ventured beyond the gate.

"Isn't it private property?" I asked.

She winked. "Nuns don't run very fast."

At recess, Beth introduced me to her best friend, Shelagh, who had blond hair like me, only longer and even curlier. They had spent grades 1 through 5 in the same class. This was the first year they'd been separated. I didn't mind sharing Beth or being the third wheel. I was happy to be part of a gang. Beth asked another girl to join us and suddenly we had a skipping group. Fifteen minutes of recess passed in seconds.

At lunchtime, I ran home to an empty house. With her diploma earned from a community college in Ontario, our mother had started to teach at Selwyn House, a private boy's school in Westmount. She was thrilled with her new job. Nancy was at Westmount High, her first day of grade 9. Lucky her, she ate lunch in the school cafeteria. I couldn't wait to indulge in french fries next year! I gobbled down my egg sandwich and left a note saying I was going to a friend's house after school.

Beth lived down the hill from us, across from Prince Albert Park. Her street was steep like ours, but the houses were smaller and grouped closer together. At the bottom of the hill, half a block away, traffic whizzed by the shops and restaurants on Sherbrooke ouest. Lucky her, living so close to the action.

"You don't have to ring the bell when you come by," Beth told me. "Friends just walk in."

Three cocker spaniels circled us as we walked into the living room, where an elderly man and woman sat on opposite ends of an ancient sofa that took up half the room. The man was reading a book. The woman was staring at her hands folded on her lap.

"Hi, Granddad. Hi, Grandma."

The old man smiled at Beth and winked at me. The old woman's head stayed bowed.

"Is your grandmother okay?" I asked, following Beth out of the room as fast as we had entered, the dogs at our heels.

"She's harmless, just a little crazy."

The grandmother was old, likely senile. I admired the way Beth brushed off a mental illness like it was nothing more annoying than an awkward piece of furniture, an oversized sofa. We continued down a narrow hall to a kitchen, barely large enough for her and me and the three cocker spaniels. I stepped on one of the tails by mistake. The counters were crammed with jars and spices. A cookbook had been left open beside the sink, which was half-full of dirty dishes. I smiled, thinking of my mother's spotless kitchen, her love of clean horizontal surfaces. Beth picked up a knife from the counter and carved a generous wedge from a pan of uncut brownies.

"My mom made these before she went to work. Help yourself, Sue." She passed me the knife.

I didn't correct her. I liked the sound of Sue. It sounded cooler than Susie or Susan.

"What does your mom do?" I already knew Beth's father lived in Australia, the farthest he could get away, she had said.

"She teaches," Beth replied.

I was about to mention that my mom was also a teacher when the basement door flew open and two boys a few years older than us stormed into the kitchen from the basement. Ignoring us, they jostled in front of the stove, carving out brownies three times the size of the ones we were eating. A trail of smoke and Pink Floyd floated up the basement stairs.

"Who's she?" the taller one asked, pointing the brownie knife at me and hoisting himself onto the counter. He looked my sister's age, pale like Beth, skinny with curly hair. I was more interested in the younger one, who hadn't yet turned around. He was wearing a denim jacket with a Rolling Stones decal on the back, half-hidden by his wavy black hair.

"We're in class together," Beth replied.

"How sweet. You good girls gonna do homework together?" said the boy with the curls, elbowing the younger one, who finally turned around. His blue eyes were a little bloodshot.

Beth sighed. "Ignore my dumb brothers. They're useless potheads."

The boys vanished into the basement, back to their smoke and music. I followed Beth and the cocker spaniels up to the second floor.

"I share a bedroom with my mom," she said, pointing at the twin beds. "It's my grandparents' house. We moved here when Dad left. It gets a little crowded at times."

I smiled. Three adults, three kids and three dogs were my kind of chaos.

She switched on the TV and flopped on the bed closest to the balcony door that overlooked the park.

"Do you have cable?" I asked.

She cocked her head. "Don't you?"

I shook mine. "We don't have colour either."

"Can't your parents afford it?"

"They can, but they're kinda weird."

"Uptight, you mean?"

"Not exactly." I pictured my mother at the piano, slapping at the keys playing boogie-woogie and my father's racy tales about life as a British naval officer. Scotch always made his stories more interesting, especially the ones about the married woman in Malta.

"It's hard to explain. They have rules."

Beth shrugged and passed me another brownie. "Take it before those idiot boys do."

We giggled and settled back in the twin beds. I hoped her younger brother would make an appearance.

"You should come for a sleepover this weekend. We can stay up late and watch movies."

This sounded like heaven.

Saturday evening, Beth's mom drove us to the A&W on rue St-Jacques in her baby blue Volkswagen Beetle. We ordered Teen Burgers and onion rings. Beth's mom allowed us to eat on the twin beds, as long as we cleaned up. I drank root beer for the first time, finishing the entire can even though it tasted a little like toothpaste. My parents disapproved of soft drinks and takeout and televisions in bedrooms. Eureka! I had struck gold!

Beth's brothers came home at ten o'clock. She and I were in the kitchen, taking turns drinking milk from the carton.

"You again," the older one said. His voice sounded hoarse.

"Better get used to it," I replied, blushing. I wondered if the younger brother had heard me. Beth was lucky. Two brothers. Sure, they teased their baby sister, but they protected her too. And brothers had friends. No boys ever turned up in our home. The only male was my father and he was a little scary.

"You look familiar," said the younger one. "Do you have an older sister at Westmount High?"

I stiffened. We didn't look the least bit alike. "Yes," I replied in a small voice. "Do you know her?"

He shrugged. "Not really."

I exhaled with relief. Nancy was not exactly a secret. I just preferred not to talk about her.

"I didn't know you had a sister," Beth said.

"We're very different. She has problems."

The younger brother guffawed. "Yeah, like I have anything in common with this little squirt." He poked Beth in the belly. "Watch out for those brownies, little sister, or you won't be little much longer."

"Stop it!" she cried, a grin on her face.

"What kind of problems?" the older brother asked.

"She's a little mental."

He popped a huge piece of brownie in his mouth.

"We know about that." He pointed to the ceiling, the grandmother's bedroom.

Beth pulled my arm. "Let's go back upstairs. I have a plan."

One warm September evening, we dragged her twin mattress to the front balcony, hung towels over the railing for privacy and made barnyard animal sounds at the people passing by on the sidewalk below. At this time of night, the streets further up the hill were empty.

"Bahhhhhh. Mooooo."

We fell back on the mattress in a fit of giggles.

Having fun wasn't the only thing Beth and I shared. By the end of the fall term, she and I were at the top of the class. In return for our good marks, Mr. Bowker turned a blind eye to the note-passing and secret sign language. His desk jumping and yelling was never directed at us. Distracted by my new friend, I was rarely at home that school year. My parents didn't protest; they were pleased with my grades, less so with my sister's performance. The illness had stolen her academic success. The studious friends she had made in grades 7 and 8 had disappeared. Frequent school absences due to doctor appointments didn't help. She was floundering.

My sister never asked for help with homework before or after her breakdown, a shame because our mother was a gifted teacher. At Mom's suggestion, I used a hot iron to press my history assignment, a letter written by a soldier fighting in the French Revolution. The burnt edges of the paper made the letter look authentically old. Mr. Bowker gave me an A+. To my surprise and delight, my mother asked me to help her grade her students' papers—a grade 4 class.

"Here's a doozie," she said, handing me a dog-eared exercise book. The handwriting was large and messy, far worse than mine had ever been.

"I can't read this!" I cried.

"Tell him so." She handed me a red pen.

I gave the assignment a C and wrote at the top of the page in neat cursive, "Repeat this exercise!"

My mother's students flooded her with gifts at the end of the school year. "Bribes from the parents," my father called them. She never sent her boys to the office; it was punishment enough for them to sit in the hall and miss her class. When someone misbehaved, she cranked the handle of the pencil sharpener attached to the blackboard and pretended to call the principal. Her theatrical performances created hysteria in the classroom. She loved to laugh, especially at fart jokes, which were rampant in a private school for boys. Some of the teachers filed complaints about my mother's rowdy class. The boys loved her. Years later, a former student introduced himself in the retirement home where our parents were living. I recognized his name from the homework assignment, the messy one. He sent me a sympathy card when my mother died, written in flourishing cursive, describing her as an important influence in his successful career as a corporate lawyer. Life may have conspired against her as a mother, but as a teacher, my mom was a shining star.

The plans I made with Beth for the Christmas holidays were cancelled when my mother was bedridden with bronchitis. I didn't mind. My mother had taken care of me so many times when I was sick; she was at her most nurturing when I was unwell. Her wet cough sounded like it was ripping her chest apart. The wastepaper basket beside the bed was full of dripping Kleenex even though I'd emptied it hours earlier. Childhood asthma had been followed by decades of smoking; her lungs would eventually kill her. That day was far in the future, the furthest thought from my twelve-year-old mind. Parents live forever. My main focus was to keep Nancy away. It was a stress my mother didn't need.

"What's Nancy doing?" my mother asked between fits of coughing.

"She's working on an assignment." It was a lie. My sister was in the kitchen foraging in the fridge. My snitching had turned to scolding; I told my sister she shouldn't leave the fridge door open for long, and why was she eating so much anyway? She ignored me, of course. I followed her upstairs, making sure she didn't disturb our mother. There was no cause for concern. Her eyes were at half-mast; the lunchtime medication cocktail had kicked in. Her room was untidy, a heap of clothes on the floor and school papers strewn over the desk. I thought about tidying.

Maybe that would help. Then my mother started coughing again.

I was making tea when the doorbell rang. The headmistress, a cur-mudgeonly, shrivelled-up spinster, stood at our front door half hidden by a pile of papers.

"Give these to your mother," she said in a piercing voice. "The grades need to be handed in this week."

How thoughtless! I wanted to slam the door on her face. I smiled politely instead.

"Also, tell her she should install a phone by her bed so she can return my calls."

Dream on, lady, I thought. A second phone? We don't even have co-lour TV.

I heaved the papers up the stairs. Nancy's door was closed.

"What did that old bat want?" my mother asked from the bed.

"She wants you to mark these papers and install a phone."

"To hell with that."

I smiled. Her feistiness was stronger than the bronchitis.

"I quit," she said.

My eyes popped open. I'd never heard of a teacher quitting halfway through the year.

"Can you do that?"

"Damn right, I can."

Unlike Beth's mother, mine didn't depend on a salary. She ignored the headmistress's threat of being blacklisted and gave a week's notice. Her boys were devastated when they heard the news. She recuperated from bronchitis and in the years to come would teach typing at a secretarial college and, later, be employed as a secretary for an Iranian carpet im-porter. Neither position came close to matching the joy she had experi-enced during her fleeting career at Selwyn House School.

My father's passion, apart from his wife, was the piano. On weekends, our house vibrated with Bach preludes and Schubert sonatas, not the most uplifting tunes for a teenager. He played the pieces over and over until he got them right—or didn't. My sister and I were lectured on the pleasure of music. To me, it looked like work: shoulders held back, fin-gers arched over the ivory keys, eyes straining to read hundreds of little black notes, the steady clicking of the metronome. Nancy sometimes sat beside him on the bench and turned the pages, although her hands were clumsier since her breakdown. Our mother didn't require sheet music.

She played old Broadway tunes from memory, one of the few things that made Norman smile.

Our father approached life with a military discipline he'd learnt as an officer in the British Royal Navy. In the short time since starting his new job with Consolidated Bathurst, he'd been promoted from senior manager to vice-president of the pulp and paper company. Despite this impressive accomplishment, his facial muscles were stuck in a grimace and he suffered from chronic insomnia.

Flurazepam helped my father sleep, amphetamines fuelled my mother and neuroleptics numbed my sister's brain. Making our household happy was more of a challenge than I'd expected. At least I didn't need psychoactive drugs to make me feel good. I had Beth and her cozy home.

Late afternoon, the same day Nancy received the "all clear" for her abdominal scan, I received a phone call from Beth, who had moved to Ontario decades earlier. She and her brothers, like the majority of Anglo-Québecers from our generation, left the province in early adulthood to pursue a career elsewhere. We lost touch for a while, but our lives intersected again when we reached middle age. Beth is one of my few friends from adolescence, which makes our relationship that much more precious. We are historic lighthouses for each other, shedding light on blurry memories—the name of the cute guy who we harassed, where we bought our first nickel bag of pot. On our call, we reminisced about all the nights I'd spent at her house across from Prince Albert Park and the irony of how I now lived so close to that home, at the bottom of the hill.

"Remember how you couldn't wait to leave Westmount?" she asked.

I laughed. But her question made me think. I had escaped Westmount around the same time that Beth moved away, but I hadn't strayed very far. Except for travel holidays, I had never left Montreal. Was I a boring homebody? Or was it because of my responsibilities? What would have happened to Nancy if I had moved away? What would have happened to me?

"Well, at least I live in Lower Westmount. I don't have to hike up a hill anymore, not unless I want to."

"Do you remember all the phone calls from your parents?"

"Which calls?"

"When they ordered you home to help with your sister."

I blanked.

"But I didn't go home, right? I stayed at your house."

She paused.

"Actually, you did go home. My mother was so upset at your parents. She said it was unfair to put the responsibility on you."

I remembered running down the hill to Beth's, nothing about going home.

"Your house was a sanctuary," I said softly. "You were lucky."

Beth laughed. "Are you kidding?"

She described her home life, the tension and challenges living with her grandmother's schizophrenia, how the stress made her grandfather sick and exhausted her mom. "It was far from a sanctuary," Beth said. My child self was shocked; a deep memory had been shifted. The adult me knew better. Every family has a story about mental illness.

"I had no idea it was that rough with your grandmother. You never complained."

"You barely mentioned your sister."

Silence. We were remembering. An incoming call on the other line brought me back to the present. Nancy. The reminder about fixing the faulty closet.

7

STANDING ON A STOOL, I INSPECTED MY FACE in the mirror of the medicine cabinet my father had hung too high. My chin was covered in microscopic dots. Blackheads, Beth called them. I ignored the tapping on the other side of the door. My sister and I shared a washroom with barely enough room for the toilet and sink, never mind two of us at the same time. The hammering of our father's morning shower in the spacious bathroom next door echoed through the common skylight. The kids' shower was downstairs in a bathroom formerly designed for a live-in maid. Why someone would need a maid in a modest-sized house like ours was ludicrous.

The tapping became more insistent.

"I need to brush my teeth," Nancy cried.

I handed her a toothbrush and re-locked the door.

"I'll tell Mom and Dad you're hogging the bathroom."

We both knew she wouldn't. Her tattling had lost authority. She was the problem daughter, not me. I opened her tube of Clearasil, dapped a spot on my chin and then wiped it off. The pink ointment stood out more than the blackheads. I opened the door slowly. Our father had retreated to the dressing room at the far end of the hall. I slipped into the parent bathroom and wiped the steam off the full-length mirror to admire my faded bell-bottoms and purple tie-dyed shirt that camouflaged my near-flat chest. The '60s were ending in three months; I was just beginning. My hair had grown below my shoulders. Still short in height and looking young for my age, at least no one would mistake me for a boy on my first day of high school.

Our parents had suggested that Nancy and I walk to school together. I had other plans. The last thing I needed was to arrive with my zombie sister who was repeating grade 9. Westmount High was a fresh start. I would meet people who didn't know my family history. Many of the Roslyn kids were attending private high schools, an option that Beth's mom couldn't afford. My parents would have paid the tuition if I had asked.

My mother was waiting by the front door. Since she had quit teaching, she had more time on her hands, too much maybe.

"What's that?" She pointed at my headband.

Beth and I had purchased matching ribbons at Miracle Mart on the metro level of Alexis Nihon Plaza. We measured the circumferences of our heads, cut the correct lengths and sewed the ends together. My mother wouldn't understand that a floral-patterned headband was an essential fall '69 accessory.

"It keeps the hair out of my face."

My mother looked skeptical.

"Why not use a pretty barrette?"

"You mean like the one Nancy wears? No thanks."

She knew better than to argue with me about fashion. I had allowed her to dress me for years, keep my hair short. Now I was in charge.

"Your sister left ten minutes ago. She's pretty slow. You can easily catch up."

I hurried down the porch steps onto the sidewalk. My mother waved her scarf from the living room window. I regretted not pausing for a proper goodbye, asking about her plans for the day. Apart from the affection between my parents, we were not a touchy-feely family. We didn't hug. Nor did we confide in each other. An unexpected jolt of sadness slowed my pace. Before Nancy's illness, my mother often let me stay home from school. She would drive us downtown and buy me a small paper bag of chocolate Rosebuds from the candy counter on the main floor of Eaton's to keep me quiet while she shopped. We ate grilled cheese sandwiches and french fries in the restaurant on the ninth floor, an art deco Montreal landmark. I was allowed to order Coke. The notes she wrote to my grades 4 and 5 teachers at Roslyn were ingenious. I loved handing them over with a straight face. *Susan had a sudden bout of nausea.* We were good company for each other. I continued down the hill towards Westmount High hoping my mother would find another job. She spent too much time alone.

Beth was waiting by the west door, where the cool older kids congregated, many of them smoking. She was in a long flowing dress her mother had made. A peace sign dangled from the silver chain around her neck.

"Did you forget your headband?" I asked.

She shrugged. "Changed my mind."

My forehead felt awkward and uncomfortable, the beginning of a headache. I pulled off the headband and shoved it in the front pocket of my jeans, next to the five-dollar bill my mother had given me for lunch.

"You don't have to take it off because I'm not wearing one."

It was my turn to shrug. "It's itchy."

Beth led us through the cloud of smokers outside the west door to the ground floor level known as the "Snakepit." She charged passed the classroom doors without reading any numbers. She knew where she was going, her older brothers' guidance. I hadn't bothered to ask my sister. I followed blindly, my stomach performing cartwheels. Thank God I wasn't alone.

Our grade 7 homeroom was a music studio. Fans of Jethro Tull, Beth and I had requested flute. I ended up with a clunky clarinet that placed me on the opposite side of the room from my friend. At lunchtime, we met up with Shelagh in the cafeteria, a cavernous space that echoed with grade 7 chatter. The cool older kids were elsewhere. My sister walked in, a paper lunch bag in her hand. She was wearing her geeky leopard-spotted pants and her hair was pulled back on one side with a brown barrette. Clearly, our mother had helped her dress. She blinked at the crowded room. I slumped down in my chair, an effort to hide. Thankfully, Nancy chose a table against the far wall. I turned the other way and bit into a soggy french fry. Cafeteria life wasn't what I had hoped for.

The next day Beth, Shelagh and I discovered the rundown triplex that the high school ran as a coffee house, destined to be demolished and replaced by my parents' future retirement home. Carrying bagels and Diet Cokes purchased at the deli across the street, we explored the three floors in search of a free corner. The students, mostly from upper grades, were sprawled over worn sofas and overstuffed chairs, too stoned to pay us any attention.

Beth nudged me. "Isn't that your sister?"

I shielded my face. "Guys, stand in front of me."

"Relax," Beth said. "She doesn't see you. Who's the guy talking to her?"

I peeked through my fingers. He was tall and skinny with long stringy hair and a matching moustache.

"Drug dealer," Shelagh whispered.

"How do you know?" I asked.

"He's way too old for high school."

I couldn't help but stare. The tall skinny drug dealer didn't hang out for long. He moved on to the next student. My sister was of no use to him. She had her own supply of pills. She sank into the depths of a bean-bag chair and closed her eyes, for a quick nap perhaps. The coffee house provided a haven for my sister. She was invisible in the smoky haze.

A few weeks later my sister discovered another refuge. As a library prefect, the nerdiest of nerdy positions, she now had the privilege of eating lunch in the library boardroom. I rarely saw her after that, except when the school was evacuated to the armoury next door. The bomb scares had nothing to do with the Front de Libération du Québec terrorists: the calls were student pranks. I looked forward to the break from class, no clue that my sister, wearing her signature blank expression, was terrified that we were about to be blown up.

At the end of grade 7, a week into summer vacation, my father called a family meeting.

"Have a seat," he told us.

Nancy flopped down beside me on the sofa. I checked my watch. A babysitting job started in ten minutes. I had earned almost enough money to buy the new James Taylor album, *Sweet Baby James*.

"What's up, Dad?" I asked.

My father stood up, never a good sign.

"We want to discuss summer plans."

"What plans?"

"Your mother and I are going to Maine and you girls are going to French camp."

Something squeezed my chest. My parents had shipped me off to Camp Kanawana the summer Nancy was first hospitalized. After one week, I'd insisted on coming home. My mother was the one to give in. I didn't "wanna" do Kanawana or any overnight camp ever again.

"I won't know anyone," I said in a sad voice.

"You have your sister."

I turned to face Nancy, curious how she was taking the news. She didn't appear the least bit upset. French camp wouldn't ruin her summer. French camp would give her a break from my parents and their shouting. My father's steel blue eyes told me there was no point in arguing. They'd already made plans for their own getaway.

Two weeks later, on the first day of camp, I found my sister's tent and joined her on the lower bunk. Her sleeping bag was still rolled up. The naked mattress felt damp and smelled like mildew. The girl above us was reading an Archie comic.

"You like it here, Nance?" I asked.

"It's okay."

She picked up a Granny Smith apple and took a bite.

"It stinks in here," I whispered.

"Insect repellent," said the girl on the upper bunk. "Your sister emptied the can."

Nancy giggled. "I'm used to weird smells."

Smells in the hospital, I thought. I wondered if anyone knew about her illness.

The next day, we exchanged glances in the dining hall. In the white T-shirt and navy shorts camp uniform, Nancy no longer stood out like she did at high school. We all looked like dorks. She strutted across the large wooden floor with her tentmates. She and the girl from the upper bunk passed by my table.

"Hey, it's your baby sister," the girl said to Nancy.

Nancy patted my head. "See you later, little sister."

She strode out of the dining hall, almost like she was normal.

The kids in my tent were friendly enough and the counsellor was lenient. I wiggled out of swimming lessons with the excuse of an earache. Nancy, meanwhile, won prizes for her crawl and butterfly. She used the money to buy a blue-and-white-striped Speedo from the camp tuck store. The bathing suit looked great on her and I told her so.

"I'm too fat," she replied and patted her belly.

Her comment was dumb, typical of what an almost sixteen-year-old girl would say. I half-listened to the boring diet she had begun to describe: iceberg lettuce, celery, cucumbers. Rabbit food. Too bad for her, she was missing out on hot dogs and ice cream and all the other food that made French camp tolerable.

The family reunited after a month sojourn. Our parents took us to an expensive French restaurant in Old Montreal. I ordered plain crêpes, the only item that appealed to me on the menu. Nancy ordered a Caesar salad without the dressing. The next morning, I was reading a detective novel at the kitchen counter while Nancy foraged in the fridge for raw vegetables. She opened and closed the cupboards. Her incessant crunching disturbed my concentration. Finally, she left. Five minutes later, a weird noise came from the maid's room bathroom. I looked up. An empty box of crackers had been left on the kitchen counter.

"You okay in there?" I called from the maid's room doorway.

"Uh-uh."

"Are you puking?"

The bathroom door opened and Nancy's face appeared.

"A cracker caught in my throat."

Two days later, I heard the same noise, this time from our bathroom upstairs.

"Another cracker?" I asked from the other side of the door.

She paused. "Yes."

I turned the door handle. Nancy was kneeling in front of the toilet. She waved me away. It didn't make sense that a cracker would make her sick. Genuinely concerned, I told my mother about the retching.

"Do you think it's the crackers?" I asked.

My mother shook her head. "Don't mention it to Nancy. Your father and I will deal with this."

The psychiatrist called my sister's condition anorexia nervosa, an eating disorder. Another round of shouting began in our home, this time about not eating enough. Perilously thin with skeletal cheekbones, Nancy was admitted to The Allan, returning full circle to where she had started. She was discharged from the hospital two months later, ten pounds heavier. Her eyelids were puffy and she smelled like Pine-Sol. She was back to Zombie Nancy. Neither my parents nor I had the patience to wait for her thoughts to be completed. It was past Thanksgiving before she was able to start grade 10.

The following spring, I was in my grade 8 music class when the office monitor knocked on our door. The teacher read, then crumpled the folded note and threw it in the garbage. She didn't take kindly to interruptions during band practice. I sympathized. The end-of-year concert was coming up fast and we still sounded pretty bad.

"Susan, you need to go to the office."

I looked over at French Horn Susan. Surely, the teacher meant her.

"Clarinet Susan!" the teacher shouted in staccato. Her baton pointed at me.

I knocked over a metal stand. Loose pages of sheet music flew into the air. I picked up the papers with shaky fingers. My marks were strong. I had done nothing wrong, except for a small incident earlier in the week. A prefect had caught me smoking in the girls' bathroom. Nothing had happened and I'd assumed the girl hadn't reported me. Until now, that is.

"Ohhhhhh, what has Susan done?" Peter Brown whispered from behind. He poked me with his trumpet. I had a small crush on Peter, who was unfortunately obsessed with Diane across the room. She had large breasts and played saxophone. I grinned at Peter, pleased with the attention.

"Naughty Susie," he said in a loud voice.

The class broke into laughter.

The teacher banged her baton on the desk.

"Settle down people, or you'll all go to the office."

We'd been together in music class for almost two years. Our poor teacher would have to endure us for another three. I forgot about the impending punishment for my smoking indiscretion and sauntered towards the door. Before leaving, I turned and bowed for my theatrical exit. The rolling laughter in the classroom carried me down the hall to the office.

The vice-principal asked me to sit in the visitor's chair. Her smile set me at ease. Perhaps I had won an award or some sort of honour that would be announced at the end-of-year ceremony. My marks were that high.

"Your mother called. She asked that you come home right after school."

"Why?" I asked, disappointed and imagining the worst.

"Your sister had some trouble today. You can leave now if you wish."

I wasn't in a hurry. Trouble was commonplace in our household. After school, I dragged my knapsack full of books onto the 124 bus that was packed with kids from Westmount High. I pushed my way through to the back and grabbed a pole. Two girls I recognized from grade 10 were sitting in front of where I stood, their legs crossed. They looked straight ahead as they talked, as if I was passing scenery.

"What's wrong with her anyway? She's so weird."

"Right? Did you hear the snores? Her head was on the desk!"

"Did you see her eyes when the teacher woke her up? It's like she had no idea where she was!"

"Crazy eyes!"

I gripped the pole. They were talking about my sister.

"She used to be an honour student."

"And now she's retarded."

I was used to smirks, whispers and stares. But the smugness of these girls on the bus really irked me.

"Excuse me," I said in the lowest, grown-up tone I could manage.

The girls looked up, their raccoon-painted eyes blank circles.

"Mental illness doesn't mean a person is retarded. Get your facts straight."

The shock on their faces started to shift to something else. My bravado waned. I hurried to the exit and leapt onto the sidewalk a stop early. My heart was still racing when the bus pulled away. I'd never defended my sister like that before. Since then, I've never stopped.

My mother was waiting on the porch. Tension etched her face. She explained that during class Nancy had become catatonic, another new word for me in my expanding sister lexicon. She had refused to leave her desk or, rather, was unable to leave. An ambulance had taken her to the Montreal General Hospital. Nancy was fine, apparently, just out of it. My mother was waiting so I could go with her to the hospital. My father was in New York making a deal to sell newsprint to some bigwig called Rupert Murdoch. I felt bad about not coming home sooner and thought better of telling her about the bus incident; she had enough on her mind. I climbed into the passenger seat and we pulled out of the driveway. Our father had traded in the Plymouth Valiant for a Pontiac Oldsmobile, a step up like his career. She drove like the wind and we arrived at the emergency in less than ten minutes. I squeezed my mother's hand, prepared to put up a fight if anyone told me I was too young to visit. Nobody did. A nurse ushered us to an examination room and closed the door. She advised us to come back in the morning; Nancy was still catatonic.

"Maybe the drugs were the problem?" I said on the drive back home.

My mother shot me a sideways look.

"Don't talk about what you don't know."

I winced but said nothing. My mother was under stress. I suggested we order takeout like we did at Beth's. My mother told me it was a waste of money. (She would have called Uber Eats "Uber Waste.")

That evening we ate ham sandwiches and watched Monty Python. I enjoyed having my mother to myself. She let me have a shower in their spacious bathroom and sleep on my father's side of the bed. I'm not sure to whom this gave greater comfort, her or myself.

I was thrilled that Sarah was coming in from Toronto for Thanksgiving, an opportunity for mother-daughter time and a break from worrying about my sister's medication. I still hadn't called her landlord about the closet that didn't slide shut. Nancy had been warned about my lack of availability over the next few days, but as often happened, my needs didn't coincide with hers. She called while I was driving home from the train station.

"I can't talk now. Just picked Sarah up," I told her.

My phone rang an hour later and an hour after that. "You're lucky you have children," Nancy yelled when I asked her to stop calling. Her voice was loaded with angry spit.

I hung up and turned off the phone. I was angry too.

Sarah and I enjoyed a relaxed dinner of sushi and sparkling white wine. At eleven o'clock, we uncurled from the living room sofa, brushed our teeth over the sink and went our separate ways to bed, me upstairs and her to the basement.

I was awake when Sarah tiptoed into my bedroom at one in the morning.

"What's up little lamb chop?"

"I heard a weird scratching sound in the wall."

"It's probably a mouse. They try to come inside this time of year."

"What if it's something bigger?"

She had inherited my worry gene. I patted the mattress.

"Snuggle up."

In her teenage years, Sarah had begged me to move her room to the basement. Now she was sleeping with me in mine. Fighting my fatigue, I reached out and touched her shoulder, careful not to wake her. Every waking moment with my daughter was precious. My eyes shone with gratitude, even in the darkness of night. Her young adult mind was healthy, beyond the age when schizophrenia usually strikes.

I imagined a different life: the terror of waking in the middle of the night and finding my thirteen-year-old daughter with the sewing scissors in her hand and a pile of blond curls lying on the floor; pinning her to the bed so the hallucinations wouldn't throw her off the balcony; the horror of leaving her on a psych ward; the heart-wrenching pain of the hospitalizations; the repeating grief.

Sarah was approaching thirty, the age when Nancy was locked away in the psychiatric hospital for thirteen years and our parents left for Germany. I would never have left the country as my mother did. I would have remained close, standing firm between my daughter and the doctors and pestering the medical staff with questions. Our mother was from an era when doctors were never challenged. She found her own way of coping with her daughter's chronic diagnosis by grabbing at the chance to live abroad with our father, to travel, paint and drink lots of wine. Her letters were always upbeat like her public persona that had attracted my father. Her dark side was more hidden, although not to us. My father, sister and I would wait for the storm clouds to blow over, never to be discussed. Who knows? Maybe my mother's flip-flop character was what helped her most to cope.

8

ELECTRODES ATTACHED TO MY SISTER'S SCALP zapped her out of catatonia. Discharged three weeks before the end of the school year, she was
too far behind to pass grade 10 biology and history, which meant repeating another year. The doctor prescribed a neutral environment to
minimize disruptions, a polite way of saying our home wasn't helping
my sister's mental health. At the beginning of September, she moved into
the Night Centre Clinic at the Reddy Memorial Hospital, one of nine
area hospitals that would eventually be closed by the Quebec government as a cost-cutting measure. Free to attend classes and come home
during the day, she checked into the clinic every evening at five o'clock.
My sister's memories of Night Centre are vague. She tells me she slept in
a dormitory where an older man repeatedly told her the same dirty joke.

What was important, Nancy says, is that she finally passed high
school. Her "Probable Destiny" caption in the 1972 yearbook reads
Becoming the first pensioner at Westmount High. At the time, I was too
young to appreciate my sister's hilarious wit that would blossom in later
years and carry us through difficult times; she refused to allow the illness
to steal her humour.

During the Night Centre phase, our house grew quiet and my parents
turned their attention to me. My buffer was gone, a loss that became apparent one warm spring Saturday evening while I was drying the supper
dishes.

"I'm going to stay at Beth's tonight," I told my mother.

She grunted. "Again?"

"It's Saturday night, Mom. I'm fourteen, not four."

"Did you do your chores?"

"Yes."

She paused. "Let me discuss with Norman."

I ran upstairs and stuffed a change of clothes and my toothbrush in a knapsack. The staircase creaked on my descent to the main floor. No magic getaway. They were waiting in the living room, Norman in his recliner, Lorna standing beside him, her hand on his shoulder. Lately, he'd been travelling less, his deals in New York concluded. I missed the cozy alone time with my mother, the relaxed rules. I slumped into the white sofa against the wall at the far end of the room, an expanse of broadloom between my parents and me. The rooms were larger without my sister in the house.

"We think you've had enough sleepovers lately. Best to stay home tonight."

"Whaaaat?"

"Your father has spoken." The frown on my mother's face aged her. She had looked younger when she was teaching.

"Beth's mother's not a good influence," my father added.

"What's that supposed to mean?"

My parents exchanged glances.

"She's a single mom," said my father.

"So what?"

"It's a wild household. No discipline."

I blinked. A wild household? Beth had a super mom. I regretted sharing the stories of eating takeout and watching television in bed, the sleepovers on the balcony. I grabbed the knapsack from the floor and stomped out of the living room.

"Come back here!" my father shouted. "How dare you walk out on us!"

"How dare you insult Beth's mom," I muttered and slammed the door behind me.

I ran to the bottom of our street and turned right. Glancing over my shoulder, a car that looked like our Oldsmobile was fast approaching. On the next block, I ducked behind the mailbox that had replaced the one blown up in 1963 by the Front de Libération du Québec. French language terrorists didn't scare me as much as my parents.

"Your mother called," Beth said when I arrived, puffing, my face beet red. "She said to call home as soon as you get here. Sounds like you're in big doo-doo."

I collapsed on their oversized sofa, close to tears.

"I hate my family."

Beth's mom appeared from the hallway.

"Do you want me to speak to them?" she asked. "Maybe I could convince them to let you stay?"

A kind offer, but one that would make them hate her even more.

My feet dragged the rest of me back up the hill. They were waiting in the living room, standing next to each other with crossed arms. I accepted their anger, no point in defending myself. It would be unkind to tell my parents that I'd left because our family home was depressing. They controlled most things but held no power over my sister's illness. Our family was doomed. I said goodnight and climbed the stairs of our joyless house.

The following September, Nancy started her two-year CEGEP program at Dawson College, located in those days down the hill from Night Centre, south of the railway tracks and the expressway. Finally freed from high school, she met a slew of new people from all over the city. The rundown campus in semi-industrial Saint-Henri suited her. She dressed in hipper clothes, made girlfriends and dated a freckled-face guy named Duncan. Fortified with independence, she whizzed through two years of college without incident, at least to my knowledge. She moved back home to prepare for university, but we rarely saw each other, except for a family holiday in Prince Edward Island pockmarked with the usual tension and blowouts caused by Nancy's refusal to conform to our parents' demands. Once again, their attention was diverted from me to her. In the span of two years, some things had changed and others not at all.

During her first year at Concordia University, my sister resided at the downtown YMCA on boulevard Dorchester, later renamed boulevard René-Lévesque. Not the trendiest address, but hugely convenient. The YMCA was across the street from Concordia's visual arts building, where Nancy spent most of her time, including weekends. University life was more stressful than college. She'd been rejected by a sorority and had fallen behind in studio assignments and the long list of required readings. Her professors were sympathetic to her illness and gave passing marks. They also recognized her talent. Not every student could sketch the human body in sixty seconds without lifting the pencil off the page.

Sunday morning, I walked past the dozing university security guard and climbed three flights of stairs. Nancy applauded when she saw me approaching from the end of the hallway. The smile on her face made me feel bad for not responding sooner to her invitations, even if we weren't in the habit of spending time together. She grabbed my hand and pulled me into the studio. The room was cluttered with easels and the air was thick with oil and turpentine. I pulled my scarf over my nose.

"Shouldn't you open a window?"

She shrugged.

"Doesn't bother me."

We stopped in front of a seated female nude painted on the rough side of a large piece of Masonite. I recognized the Matisse style from a piece hanging in the Musée des beaux-arts de Montréal—intense colour, undulating contours and decorative pattern. The nude figure, painted magenta and ochre, resonated against a background of greens and blues. The figure's legs and arms felt deliberately out of proportion compared to the oversized head and torso. The face, expressionless with a fixed, unwavering gaze, made me shiver. The painting was beautiful.

"Who painted this?"

My sister laughed. "Me, silly."

My attention returned to the woman's face. "Was she a model?"

"She's a compilation of you and me."

The watery eyes and turned-up nose belonged to my sister. The generous mouth and strong chin were mine. The body belonged to neither of us.

I glanced at the neighbouring easels belonging to the other students: a vase with flowers, snowcapped mountains, a dog's happy face. The small brushwork detail in these paintings had taken hours to create. My sister's flat and loose strokes were feathery and light, with a rushed quality like a bird's wings in flight. Except for the face.

"How long did this take to paint?"

She hesitated. "Forty-five minutes."

"Wow. Do you paint that quickly all the time?"

"I do things my way."

I didn't ask what the professor had said about that.

"I have zero patience for small brushes," she added.

I was impressed. This was a rebellious side I had never seen before, apart from her behaviour with my parents.

Our next stop was the ceramic studio. Nancy showed me several pieces she'd made in pottery class: a coil pot painted two shades of blue; a shallow dish with a bumblebee engraved in the centre; a ceramic apple strudel; the face of a psychiatrist with pencil-thin lips and gaping large eyes; a pistol with a cloud painted on the side with the figure nine.

"Make something," she said, handing me a slippery clump of clay.

"Are you serious? I can't do art."

She reached for a small sculpture on the shelf.

"Copy this," she said. "It's not difficult."

I rolled the clay into a ball, not taking my eyes off the Romanesque torso she'd placed in front of me. I worked quickly. My fingers prodded and squeezed to form upper thighs, a protruding belly, small breasts and sloping shoulders. The final product, to my surprise, looked like a torso.

"Beginner's luck," Nancy muttered.

She had no need to be jealous; Nancy had found her passion. Mine was nowhere to be seen. I thanked her for the studio tour and retraced my steps down the third-floor hall towards the stairwell.

The next morning I intercepted my father on his way out the front door.

"Dad, I need to talk to you about something."

He set down his briefcase. The grimace across his face, more pronounced than usual, warned me that my timing was off.

"You're still planning on going to university?" he asked.

I chortled, a nervous response.

"I won a scholarship, remember? It would be a waste not to use it. And all that money you spent on my college tuition."

Unlike Nancy, I had insisted on attending a private CEGEP, Marianopolis College, known for high academic standards. My father's grimace deepened even further, a signal to get to the point.

"So . . . should I apply to the McGill management program or . . ."

"Or what?"

I shrugged. "Dunno. Maybe study music?"

"Music? You haven't played the clarinet in over two years."

"I could pick it up again."

"You can't just put down and pick up an instrument."

"What about an arts degree?"

His right eyebrow lifted. "What would you do with that?" he asked.

"Don't have a clue. That's why I'm asking."

He paused.

"It's up to you," he said, picking up his briefcase. "Are you planning on coming up north with us this weekend?" Up north was a cottage my parents had built in the Laurentians; a refuge in the Canadian wilderness was our father's dream. Thick woods enveloped the cedar-shingled house located five miles down a sparsely populated dead-end dirt road. My sister didn't mind the isolation. I hated it. At seventeen, separation from friends was pure torture. Constant complaining about cottage life had weakened my parents' resolve; for the past year, they'd allowed me to stay solo in the city.

"No, I'm staying here, remember? Mom said I could host a small gathering at the house."

He grunted and then he was gone, leaving me alone at the open front door. I blinked at the morning light, confused by my father's mixed message. Music was no longer an option according to him. My suggestion of an arts degree had not gone over well. But he had said it was up to me. I had hoped for a more in-depth discussion. I had a solid music background and my English literature grades were high. We hadn't even discussed where the management program might lead. Seeing as I had no clue what to study, management seemed as good an option as any. Surely, my father would be pleased I was following in his business footsteps.

Five months had passed since the sticky July afternoon when I'd accompanied my sister to her appointment at the External Clinic for Psychotic Disorders. We were now in freezing December. Nancy called me in the late morning, elated. The gradual lithium reduction closely monitored by Dr. Byrne was over. She had taken her last pill. Finally, the shaking had eased off! We made plans to meet at the food court in Alexis Nihon Plaza. She had a craving for an all-dressed pizza.

The mall was draped in garish Christmas décor, suitably festive for our celebratory meeting. I rode the escalator to the food court floor. A homeless woman was sleeping at one of the tables next to the atrium in the spot where Nancy and I were meant to meet. I looked around for my sister, who arrives at appointments pathologically early. I checked the pizza counter and the stalls in the women's washroom, then returned to the atrium. My breath caught in my throat when I recognized the turquoise eyeglass frames on the table beside the homeless woman's sleeping head. I rushed over.

"Nancy, are you okay?" I asked, touching her arm. Her sweater was soaked with sweat and she was trembling, even without lithium.

"You're burning up. Are you sick?"

"No."

"What's going on?"

She moaned.

"What can I do?"

"Nothing."

"Should I get help?"

"No."

Her eyelashes fluttered like she was dreaming. Unpleasant memories resurfaced of the adolescent zombie and, later, her bad days on the locked ward. I slumped down in the chair beside her. This is what my sister looked like off lithium. I felt horribly responsible—my persistent suggestions to reduce the dosage without realizing that the side effects were a small price to pay for stability. I stroked a lock of her hair, unsure what to do. She had told me to do nothing, not to get help. My heart ached from her suffering, the wide-awake nightmare.

Thirty minutes later, Nancy's eyes opened. She pushed up to sitting, retrieved a plastic water bottle from one of her shopping bags, drank the contents within seconds and reached for her coat.

"Let's go!" she said, standing up.

"Go where?" I asked blinking.

"Shopping! I need socks and underwear. Look at all those Christmas lights. So bright and twinkly. We should buy some for my balcony. Can we do that? I'm hungry. Let's get some pizza. But first, I have to pee."

Her speech was rushed and breathy. She wasn't complaining or giving me a hard time. She was in an uncharacteristically pleasant mood, elated like she had sounded during our phone call that morning. Her eyes were shining. Her hands, no longer trembling, moved freely as she rattled on. The chatter was a relief, but disconcerting.

I pulled at her arm. "Sit down a sec, Nance. Take it easy."

She shook me off.

"I don't need to take it easy, thank you. I'm fine."

She stumbled away from the table at a remarkably quick pace for someone who had emerged from a catatonic stupor. I hurried to catch up. Zombie sister had morphed into polite speedy sister, a new twist.

We ordered pizza, but I didn't have time to finish mine; Nancy was already on the go. She rushed out of the food court, up the escalator and into Winners. Her usual crooked gait had straightened a little. She snapped up a three-pack of ankle socks without examining the package as she usually would and headed for the checkout with me trailing behind, queasy from the combination of worry and food-court pizza. We parted ways at the store entrance.

The walk along boulevard de Maisonneuve was steadying, even if the air was bloody cold. Late afternoon, the sun was already dipping below the horizon. Winter had arrived, the first one since Keith and I had stopped migrating to Costa Rica. Halfway home, I pulled out my phone and left a message for Dr. Byrne, alerting him about my sister's dramatic mood swing. I refrained from calling Keith at the cottage and dumping on him. My disappointing news about Nancy's condition could wait.

Arriving home, I kicked off my leather boots and headed for the kitchen. The fridge was barren. I didn't feel like schlepping groceries; instead, I collapsed on the sofa in my unzipped coat and stared at the ceiling. An hour later, my grumbling stomach woke me. I grabbed the car keys, pulled on my boots and headed into the evening in search of a meal. I turned down the Glen and sailed into Saint-Henri. It felt good to get out of Westmount.

Thursday night marks the beginning of a Montreal weekend. Bars and restaurants are notoriously busy, even at six o'clock. Fortunately, a parking spot was available across from a trendy Mexican eatery on rue Notre Dame. Even luckier, a place was available at the bar. I slipped into the seat across from the bartender, who was spearing three giant olives onto a long toothpick that he dropped into a bird-bath-sized martini glass. He caught me staring.

"Would you like one?" he asked.

Tempting, but I was driving. I ordered a glass of Pinot grigio and a plate of nachos and turned to survey my surroundings. The restaurant was packed with twenty-somethings too busy with themselves and each other to notice a much older woman seated at the bar. The invisibility was a delightful escape from my day. The bartender presented the Pinot grigio with a wink. I took a long and slow sip. The youthful chatter around me was full of enthusiasm. I swivelled playfully on the bar stool and straightened my slouched back.

"Sue?"

Years had passed since I'd seen Willy's high-school friend Zachary. At twenty-six, he had grown tall.

"Where's Keith?" Zach asked, eyeing the young men sitting on either side of me.

"At the cottage. I'm here for a quick bite. Too lazy to cook."

"Sweet. Hey, I hear Will's working on a TV series."

"Yup. His camera work has finally gone legit."

The bartender grabbed the edge of the bar with his long tattooed arms and leaned towards me. "You know Zach?" he asked.

"Know him? I practically raised him."

Zach patted my shoulder. "Sue is Will's mom."

The bartender studied my face. His eyes lit up when he recognized the strong mother-son resemblance.

"I can tell," he said grinning.

So much for invisibility.

"What are you up to?" I asked, pointing at the tripod poking out of Zach's knapsack.

Zach glanced over at the two twenty-something males at a nearby table.

"We're on a mission," he said.

"Where are you headed?" I asked, lowering my voice.

"An old factory on William."

I pointed at the duffle bag on the floor.

"You have lots of gear."

"We're setting up a time-lapse on the roof. It'll take hours."

The server appeared at their table with a tray full of food.

"Bon appetit!" I said.

I swivelled back to the bar where a plate of steaming nachos had been delivered and inhaled the fresh tomato and melted Monterey Jack, suddenly ravenous. Twenty minutes later, my plate was clean and my glass was empty. I flagged the bartender for the bill.

"Have fun on your mission," I said, patting Zach's shoulder.

"It's not happening," one of his friends replied.

"How come?"

"Our driver crapped out on us."

I hesitated.

"Can I give you guys a lift?"

They brightened, revealing little boy smiles behind their facial hair.

"Awesome," Zach said.

"Maybe I could go inside, just for a few minutes, if that's okay? I love old factories."

Zach glanced at his friends. They shrugged.

"Sure," he said.

The boys followed me out of the restaurant and into my car. En route to our destination, Zach and I reminisced about Will's urban exploring adventures. The two friends listened in the back seat, fascinated or maybe shocked by the stories a mother was sharing. I parked between lampposts half a block from the defunct factory. The boys grabbed their knapsacks, adjusted the straps on their shoulders and hurried towards a broken section of steel fencing. I surveyed my boots. Italian leather.

"Hmm, not sure about that fence, guys."

"Just be careful where you plant your feet and look out for barbed wire."

They made it sound easy. I hovered on the sidewalk, unsure. Approaching headlights turned my head. A police cruiser was creeping towards us.

"Cops!" I shouted. "You guys go on. I'll deal with it."

Zach and his friends disappeared into the shadows. The cruiser pulled up to where I was waiting on the sidewalk. The window lowered. I was the first to speak. "Good evening, officer. Have you seen a ginger tabby? Someone reported my missing cat on William, which is strange since I live miles away in Lower Westmount. Then again, cats wander." The officer smiled and told me I should be careful; this was a rough neighbourhood. I pointed my keys at the Audi and assured her I didn't plan on staying.

I collapsed in the driver's seat, heart fluttering from the adventure. My phone lit up: Nancy—a sign she wasn't catatonic. I didn't feel like answering. The call would kill the adrenaline rush, as small as it was. My sister didn't approve of her nephew's urban exploring, just as she had pooh-poohed my childhood escapades. She still scolded me for my adult antics, like buying a house in Costa Rica. Was this straight side of her a way to control me? Or a way to control her illness? What if she had a healthy mind? Would she climb to the roof of this abandoned factory, settle beside me in front of a vent and dangle her feet over the metal flashing? I would love nothing more than to show her the night city sky, how the cross on Mount Royal glows with phosphorescent white and the houses in Upper Westmount twinkle like a thousand stars. We would huddle under the throw blanket she'd woven, close our eyes and allow the city sounds to calm us, neither of us anxious nor angry. We would no longer be mad sisters.

The headlights from the police cruiser flashed on and off, a signal for me to move on. I pulled away from the curb and wished the boys well. Twelve minutes later, I was home.

9

AT THE TIME OF MY INDECISION about university, I was straddling two different friend groups: a tight gang of Marianopolis College students destined for professional careers and a loose circle of urban bohos I'd met through my recent friend, Libby, whom I'd first encountered at five in the morning following my high school grad party. I was in Murray Hill Park at the time, playing Frisbee with a dozen other still-tipsy graduates. A dark figure strolled across the baseball field towards us. The face was hidden in the shadow of a hood attached to a long velvet black cape that dragged across the dewy grass. "It's the Grim Reaper!" someone shouted and the game came to a standstill. I was convinced one of the football jocks had dressed up as a prank. The figure walked up to where I was standing and removed the hood, revealing a long mane of thick red hair. It was Libby, the new girl from Vancouver who'd arrived halfway through grade 11. I'd heard she was a gifted painter. She greeted me in the same friendly manner as Beth on our first day of grade 6. I asked Libby if she wanted to play. She said she preferred to sit and watch. Did I want to join her? We sat cross-legged on the damp grass, shared a cigarette and watched the sunrise. I was certain Libby's arrival at the dull Frisbee game was a good omen.

Libby was the first person I invited to the party. Saturday evening, on the heels of the brief university conversation with my father, my parents' house was rocking. Many of the revellers were friends of friends. Party crashing was common practice, especially in the boho circle. I'd done it myself. The electric crowd mingled thanks to the mound of marijuana and chunks of hash on the dining room table, courtesy of a Marianopolis friend with wealthy parents. I retreated upstairs to the den with a junior pro tennis player I'd met in my college economics class. My mother called him a drowned rat. A former boyfriend (we'd broken off that afternoon) stormed into the den where the rat and I were holding hands on the loveseat. A stoned altercation ensued. The tennis player ran off for fear of a broken wrist and I made my way to the bathroom to re-adjust my outfit—tight white jeans and a white halter top.

My heart was still racing from the kerfuffle when I re-entered the den. My former boyfriend was fiery but not unreasonable. The damage was minimal: one thrown pillow, a knocked-over lamp and a shattered light bulb. The couple who'd taken over the loveseat didn't seem to notice. I descended into the cloud of smoke on the main floor. Libby was sitting on the stairwell landing with a geeky-looking guy I'd seen at a couple of parties, a neighbour of hers. She invited him to all the events. She was sweet that way.

"Did you know your sister is here?" she asked me.

I did not.

Nancy was leaning against the fridge talking to an older man and woman I didn't recognize. I tapped my sister on the shoulder.

"You're supposed to be at the cottage with Mom and Dad," I shouted above the noise.

She leaned closer. Her hair smelled earthy and her eyes were bloodshot. I'd never seen her stoned before, on recreational drugs, that is. As far as I knew, she didn't go to parties. Our parents would freak if they knew. Pot didn't mix well with antipsychotics. She waved her arms in the air.

"You call this a small gathering?"

"I won't tell Mom and Dad if you don't."

"Oh, they'll find out."

I knew what she meant. The smoke alone would take hours to clear, even with the doors and windows open. I opened the fridge and grabbed a Labatt Blue.

"Want one?" I asked.

She shook her head and grabbed the arm of the older man.

"This is Stéphane, my drawing professor."

The professor looked early thirtyish. His dark curly hair was pulled back in a ponytail and he had a small goatee. The woman leaning on him was dressed all in white like me; only she wore a low-cut peasant dress tied tight around her slim waist with a leather belt.

"And his wife," she added.

"I have a name," the woman replied with a slurry voice. "Marie-France."

The wife looked me up and down. "Do you have anything strong to drink?"

"Just beer." No way would I share my tequila with a drunken stranger.

Marie-France opened the fridge. "Ohhh, I love Camembert!"

Nancy and I exchanged glances. Our father's favourite cheese.

"What's up with the professor's wife?" I whispered.

"I didn't know he was married," she replied evenly.

I knew my sister was disappointed. The professor was kind of cute.

"The cops are here!" someone cried out.

"Bravo!" cried Marie-France. "Maybe they'll liven up this party."

With "Love Machine" blaring in the background, I assured the policeman the music would be turned down. On my way to the stereo, I was intercepted by a drummer I'd met through Libby. Reminiscent of a young De Niro, he was a welcome replacement for the junior tennis pro. We headed upstairs, leaving my sister, the cute professor and his thirsty-hungry wife behind.

An hour later, I couldn't find Nancy or her friends. The wife, to my horror, was on the back porch swilling back my father's single malt Scotch whisky. I toured the main floor and returned upstairs. A low moaning led me to our parents' walk-in closet. I banged my fist on the door.

Exit the professor, looking sheepish, with his half-baked schizophrenic drawing student in pursuit. I gave the prof a dirty look. Shame on him. He left the party soon after with a drunken Marie-France in tow. Nancy sank into the living room sofa and closed her eyes. "Bohemian Rhapsody" was blasting from our father's Bose speakers. The hand-woven carpet was littered with potato chips and cigarette ash. An ocean of empty beer bottles, many of them fallen over, covered our parents' beloved teak coffee table. Meanwhile, the drummer was waiting upstairs. I collapsed on the sofa beside my sister, exhausted and overwhelmed.

"Can you call me a cab?" she asked. Her eyes were half-open.

The back of my jeans felt strangely damp. I pushed up to standing, exposing a blood stain on the white sofa. My period had arrived early.

"Hold on," I told her. "I gotta change before I call your taxi."

I ran out of the room before she had a chance to object. The party was over, at least for my sister and me.

Four o'clock in the morning, I started the deep clean. One guest remained: Libby's neighbour, who had passed out on the stairway landing. I poked him with a toe.

"Time to hit the road, Jack."

"It's Paul, not Jack," he moaned.

I turned on the vacuum. Paul reached for the banister, a drunken smirk on his face. I remembered the tequila shots and how he'd tried to kiss me. The memory, combined with the clinking of broken glass being sucked up the vacuum hose, made me queasy. An hour later, I was wiping down the teak coffee table when Paul staggered out the door. I continued to tidy and clean, all the while cursing my friends who were sleeping off their hangovers in the comfort of a bed.

My parents' car pulled into the driveway at noon.

"What's that smell?" my mother asked, her nose lifted in the air.

"What smell?"

She walked into the dining room, which had been a hash den hours earlier. Her eyes dropped to the table.

"What's that?" she asked, pointing at a minuscule mark on the finish.

I scanned the room. Someone had turned one of the paintings upside down. I prayed she wouldn't notice.

"How many friends were here?"

"Fifteen," I lied.

"Did you consume alcohol?"

"There was some beer."

"Any drugs?" My mother was sniffing again.

"Some kids smoked pot."

"Did you smoke?"

"No," I lied again.

Sleep-deprived with a tequila hangover, I couldn't handle an inquisition.

"So, what's my punishment?"

My mother looked me up and down, more from curiosity than anger.

"You look awful. Go get some sleep."

I dragged myself up the staircase and paused on the landing to pick up a beer cap. The party had been a success, but at what cost? The neighbour who called the cops would surely complain to my parents and tell them about the sixty people they'd seen entering the house. I needed to replace an expensive bottle of Scotch. And the cheese. Nobody had stayed to help me clean and a horny drawing professor had taken advantage of my sister. Clearly, fun and responsibility didn't mix.

"I'll never host another party in this house," I shouted down at my parents.

Twelve hours later, I slinked downstairs, starved. Midnight, my parents were asleep. A wedge of quiche had been left for me in the fridge. In the morning, neither parent mentioned the party or the punishment. For the next twenty-four hours, I roamed the house with extreme caution, chastising myself for not knowing better. If I wanted to have a good time, I'd need to venture farther than the family home.

Shortly after the house party, Nancy moved back home; she'd been caught with a man at the YWCA, the professor perhaps. The reintegration into our rigid family life, combined with the pressure of university triggered her agitation. Her yelling and swinging limbs never resulted in physical violence, but the verbal assaults were disturbing. I avoided home and my stormy sister as much as possible; I had my own pressures.

I tapped lightly on the door before entering my sister's bedroom. She was nestled in a beanbag chair, a spiral-bound drawing pad on her lap and a box of charcoal at her feet. Ripped-out sketches were scattered across the floor. She looked up at me, her eyes narrowing.

"Can I help you?" she asked.

"I want to talk to you about something."

"What?"

"How did you end up studying fine arts?"

"It was Mom's idea."

I scanned the paintings our mother had hung on my sister's bedroom walls, including the Matisse-like seated nude I'd admired in the studio. Nancy's eyes were on mine, reading my mind as she often does.

"I'm sure you didn't need anyone to tell you what to study. You'll have an important career, just like Dad." Her voice was screwed tight with resentment.

"You don't know me very well," I said.

She picked up a piece of charcoal from the box and waved it at me, as if mapping out my portrait.

"*Au contraire*, dear little sister. I know you very well."

Her hand glided over the sketchpad, filling the blank page with black swirling lines until a face appeared. Conversation over, I returned to my room and shoved *Basic Economics* by Thomas Sowell into my weighted knapsack. What would our mother have suggested if I had approached her for advice instead of our father? Would she have said it was up to me? Or would she have encouraged my interest in the arts? Too late, I was halfway through my first year at McGill, already fatigued by auditorium lectures, statistical formulas and briefcase-carrying students obsessed with grades. My boho friends repeatedly asked why I'd chosen a field I so disliked. My answer was always the same: a sheepish shrug. I didn't tell them that I'd made a mistake. Fortunately, I'd discovered the perfect antidote for my management school blues.

Unknown to my family, I paid Libby a small rent to sleep at her apartment on the weekends. She'd moved out of her parents' Westmount house to the second floor of a greystone triplex on Lambert-Closse, a block east of Atwater and a gateway to downtown. Her living room window was in the shadow of the Montreal Forum and diagonally across from the infamous twenty-four-hour Moe's Snack Bar, where we often ate breakfast before falling in bed after an extended night. Libby had a talent for picking up stray people; her apartment had become a mecca for musicians, poets, painters, writers and the unemployed. Moving between my different worlds was a tricky transition, yet somehow, I'd managed to maintain a 3.8 grade point average, not bad considering 4 was a perfect score. Maybe my sister was right: maybe business was my destiny.

Sunday evening, I rushed up Lambert-Closse, turned onto Sherbrooke and entered the tree-lined streets of Westmount. In ninety minutes, our friends' band would be playing at the John Bull, a dimly lit pub off a concrete tunnel that ran between Drummond and Stanley, a tunnel that no longer exists. If I moved fast enough, there would be just enough time to pick up a change of clothes at my parents' house and head downtown in time for the first set.

I marched through the front door and saluted my father in his leather recliner. He raised his hand and returned to the papers he was reading, probably work stuff, given the open briefcase next to his slippered feet. My mother was in the upstairs den, bent over the ironing board. I poked my head through the doorway and asked how she was.

"Not great," she replied in a voice I could barely hear, especially with the television blaring.

"How come?"

She sprayed the shirt collar with starch and picked up the iron.

"I'm sick of this," she said.

"Why don't you take a break?"

"Your father needs five shirts for his week."

"Can't they just drip dry?"

She glared at me, a signal to back off.

"What did you eat today?" she asked.

"Souvlaki."

She screwed up her face. "I smell garlic."

The iron hissed over my father's collar. Four more wrinkled shirts were waiting in a heap at the end of the ironing board. The fake laughter from the sitcom was depressing. I couldn't wait to get away.

"I'm going back to Libby's. Back tomorrow after class."

"Did you check in with your father?"

"Yes."

I gave her a quick peck on the cheek and ran to my room for fresh clothes.

"You're leaving?" my father asked, lowering his papers as I snuck past the living room. The creaky floorboards had betrayed me again.

"I'll be back tomorrow."

"Come closer."

I took a step forward. The glare from the 100-watt lighting was blinding.

"What's wrong with your eyes?" he asked, studying my face.

"It's bright in here."

"You're becoming a night owl."

He had a point. My sleep routine was wonky.

"Where are you going?"

"Libby's."

"That's idiotic. Do you realize what time it is?"

"My accounting class doesn't start until noon."

"You're wasting your time hanging out with that slovenly slut."

My cheeks burned. I knew what he was thinking: that I stayed at Libby's so I could have sex with whomever and whenever I wanted. He couldn't be more wrong. My boho friends teased me about being uptight and shy. They joked about my phantom chastity belt. They didn't know me any better than my parents did, at least not from a sexual perspective.

I enjoyed sexual intimacy; I just wasn't interested in one-night stands.

"Libby is not a slut," I muttered.

"Lebbie Libby," my father hissed.

My chin raised high, I swung around, stormed into the living room and came to a halt two feet from my father's icy stare. These were not the same "baby blues" described in his Scotch-induced stories about how he'd batted his eyelashes to get free entrance to the cinema or a free pint from the barmaid. That playful youth had been replaced by a hardened, middle-aged man who worked long hours in a stressful job he didn't like and whose daughters were a big disappointment. I wondered what else had gone awry in his life.

"I'm eighteen years old, Dad. I can go where I want."

I waited with fisted hands for his rebuttal. Nothing. Only the icy stare. I hesitated, unsure, and glanced down at his wristwatch. Thirty minutes before the band's set would start. I hurried to the front door and ran into the night, which for me had just begun.

Once again on lithium, Nancy stabilized within a week. We were back where she'd started before the gradual reduction, except the catatonia still randomly resurfaced for an hour or two. That happens, Dr. Byrne told us. Nancy's shaking also returned, as did her frustration. Once more, our conversations were sharp with jabs and complaints. My sister and I were back to duelling.

"Dad used to tell me things," she told me over the phone.

"Nancy darling, I'm sure he did," I replied, half-listening. "He told me things too."

"I'm talking about private matters."

"Like what?" I replied, irritated by her superior tone.

"He once told me that he'd married the wrong woman."

I rolled my eyes. "Come on, Lorna and Norman were inseparable. Once she was gone, Dad hung in for only three months."

"It's true. He said so."

"When?"

"In the hospital."

I didn't trust her memory—shock therapy and all those drugs. "Which hospital? When exactly?"

"The Douglas. They were visiting from Germany. I was thirty-one."

"Are you sure?"

"Of course, I'm sure. He said he regretted marrying Mom."

"Why would he tell you and not me?"

"Darling, like I said, he told me things."

Nancy could have been making the story up to make me jealous, another one of her jabs. Then again, maybe she was telling the truth. This could explain why he was so miserable. Our father was not exempt from our mother's temper. She'd lain into him full throttle during her amphetamine withdrawal and, later, he bore the burden of her dementia. It pained me to see him so diminished in the retirement home, so dependent on my visits. In that last year, I suspected the cancer had come back. No more doctors, he'd insisted. I'd hoped to spend time with him after our mother passed, but he was skin and bones, nothing left. I'll never know if he thought he'd married the wrong woman. All he ever talked to me about was investments and banking.

10

IN 1976, ON THE FIFTEENTH OF NOVEMBER, independence activist René Lévesque was elected premier of Quebec, thereby triggering a long exodus of anglophones who feared their province would secede from Canada. Housing prices in Montreal plummeted, Westmount included. Norman and Lorna Grundy were not the least bit threatened by the possibility of Quebec sovereignty. In fact, they admired René Lévesque's abrupt manner and choleric defence of his ideals. So, it surprised me when a For Sale sign appeared on our front yard in the spring of 1977. My father explained that he wished to downsize to a simpler life downtown, which confused me as well. Mid-fifty seemed young for downsizing. Our house, priced low, sold quickly. My parents had accepted the first offer, a decision that made no business sense. Only later did I understand how desperate they were for change.

I took a break from packing, stepped onto the balcony and inhaled the spring air. I had moved into my sister's room during her month-long hospitalization following an unfortunate accident at the pet store where she had cleaned the mice cages and left the doors open. (Nancy later confided that she'd felt imprisoned by her summer job and family life.) Back from the hospital and in her final year of studio arts, she had been indifferent about the switch of bedrooms, just as she didn't care about our impending move. Experience had taught her that living arrangements were often temporary.

My mother was on the deck below, hanging damp sheets. She was whistling an old Broadway tune, one of the pieces she played on the piano. The grey tabby from next door, now a geriatric cat, sauntered into the yard and rubbed against her bare leg. She scolded the cat in the loving tone reserved for our father. I leaned over the railing. Cut lilacs had been carefully arranged in the garden basket beside the laundry hamper. There would be no flowers or backyard where we were headed. I turned from the balcony and stepped into the bedroom. Nancy was at an art history class and our father was in Europe on business. My mother needed my help. I would box my belongings and then move on to my sister's, just as Nancy had packed up my Etobicoke bedroom ten years earlier.

Our parents had signed a lease with the Port-Royal Apartments on Sherbrooke ouest, in the Golden Square Mile district, formerly an enclave of Montreal's Anglo elite. Thirty-three storeys high, the Port-Royal was the highest residential building in Montreal and would remain so for another sixteen years. Our new residence was on the nineteenth floor, no balcony and windows that were kept closed on account of the whistling draft from the strong winds off the mountain. A fortress. Our parents had enticed me with my own entrance, bedroom and bathroom, rent-free. In return, I would have to commit to a full year. We never discussed why they were so adamant that their almost twenty-year-old daughter should move with them. I assumed they were clinging to a semblance of family and that they needed my help with Nancy. With two semesters remaining in the management program, it made financial sense to accept their offer.

Six months later, on a Sunday night, Libby and I smoked a joint on her black leatherette sofa and listened to Fleetwood Mac's *Rumours*. Two friends turned up and we piled into a taxi that delivered us to the Palace Theatre, where we watched David Lynch's new film *Eraserhead*, a welcome change from *The Rocky Horror Picture Show*, which we'd seen a zillion times. The bland factory life of *Eraserhead*'s hero, Henry Spencer, made my hands sweat and my heart beat fast. My future looked equally dull as his. The second joint we'd smoked in the taxi hadn't helped.

We poured onto Ste-Catherine ouest and checked a friend's answering machine, a valuable source of information on "happenings," which were dutifully recorded every evening, even on Sundays—a late '70s version of posting on Facebook. Our ears perked up at the description of a party in the Mile End. We hailed a taxi, two bottles of cheap Spanish Rioja between the four of us. The host was a film director, according to Libby. He greeted us in his crowded hallway, over fifty and balding, wearing a black shirt that exposed a hairy grey chest and a heavy gold chain. An hour later (or was it two?), he was posing under a Frank Zappa poster in his kitchen when he caught my stare.

"What's your name?" he asked, pulling the strap of my tank top back onto my narrow shoulder.

I hesitated; *Susan* sounded ordinary.

"Susie Cream Cheese," Libby replied.

The name came from a Zappa song, a reference to a group of Jewish girls, fans of the Mothers of Invention who'd promoted the band, danced at the front of their gigs to get the crowds going and likely performed other services. The film director's smile revealed a set of stained, crooked teeth. His eyes, narrow slits, studied my face.

"How old are you, Susie Cream Cheese?"

His soft, hoarse voice gave me unpleasant shivers. I wavered. He turned away, not waiting for my answer. At twenty, I looked seventeen.

We stayed at the party until four in the morning. The third taxi of the evening carried us back across town to Libby's apartment on Lambert-Closse. Our group had expanded from four to six. Somehow, we had all crammed into the cab.

"Moe's, anyone?" asked Libby.

An early October dawn strained through the dusty windows at Moe's Corner Snack Bar. Moe had a loyal following of Hollywood actors, Montreal Canadiens hockey players, taxi drivers, cops, bartenders, writers, musicians, painters and prostitutes. I broke off a piece of toast and soaked up the remains of the bacon and eggs that Moe Sweigman himself had served. Uprooted from Halifax, he'd bought the diner in 1958. "Say it ain't so, Moe," *Montreal Gazette* journalist John Meagher would write in 2015, lamenting the loss of the "time-capsule" diner when Moe announced his retirement.

"Want that last piece of toast?" Libby asked.

I pushed my plate towards her. The two guys across from us in the booth were watching closely, still hopeful even at five o'clock in the morning. We'd been unable to shake them off at the Mile End party. The one across from me was not bad-looking. He had said he worked in a bookstore; I couldn't remember which one.

Mary Sawyer appeared at the end of our booth, a burning cigarette between her teeth and eyes on the two guys. Her schizophrenia had surfaced later than Nancy's, at nineteen instead of thirteen. Unlike my sister,

Mary oozed with confidence. She spoke with a slurry smoker's voice and dressed in expensive hip clothes and silver jewellery, often with someone on her arm.

"Who are these two sweeties?" she asked.

I stood up to pay.

"Take my seat, Mary."

"Where ya going?" asked the not-bad-looking guy.

"If I don't get home before daylight, I'll turn into a potato."

I winked at Libby and walked over to the cash. I missed the convenience of the one-minute walk from Moe's to her couch, but I needed a good sleep.

The overcast sky matched the grey concrete of the Montreal Forum, now called the Old Forum by some, and the AMC Cinema by others. Our "Habs" would win ten Stanley Cups over the eighteen years Moe owned the diner. He was their good-luck charm. My love affair with hockey had been brief: a blind date with a Habs forward set up by a disc jockey at CKGM Radio, where I worked as a part-time researcher during my last year at university. My hockey player had been hit in the mouth by a puck. "A stitchy kisser," I told Libby. The relationship was fleeting. Apart from being born in Ontario, we had nothing in common.

Sober and spent, I climbed the four steps between Moe's and the sidewalk and turned east. A biting wind pushed me forward. I zipped up my black leather jacket and continued along the deserted high-rise corridor. My boot heels clicked past the dry cleaners, the pizza restaurant, the police station. I turned left at Concordia University's Hall Building, a prefabricated, stressed concrete cube in the style of the brutalist movement, according to Nancy. Over the summer, she completed her arts diploma at Concordia, and last month, she entered the master's program in art education at McGill. She missed the structure and security of the studio. The new program was unnerving and failed to ground her. The day before, she had freaked out at a silverfish in our parents' bathroom. The screams were heard from the elevator. Not a good sign.

The white stone pillars of the Port-Royal fortress were glowing, even on a dull autumnal morning. I reached for the polished brass handle. The glass door flew open, powered by Giovanni, the doorman. We nodded at each other. In the six months following our family's move, Giovanni and I had rarely exchanged words, yet he had witnessed my comings and goings and my strange acquaintances, including a drunken poet who'd followed me home as far as the door. The next evening, the poet somehow skipped past Giovanni's surveillance and rang my buzzer at midnight, unaware that I lived with my parents, a detail I had not mentioned. My father's face had turned a striking purple. He was not a fan of poets, drunken or sober.

Giovanni disappeared as the elevator doors clicked shut. In an hour, the residents of the Port-Royal, including my father, would be riding down to the lobby in suits with briefcases headed for the office. I would be sound asleep. The elevator released me on the nineteenth floor. The plush carpeting muffled my boot heels and I slipped through my private entrance like a well-oiled key. My boots, jacket and jeans flew in the direction of a chair, and I fell into bed, exhausted.

I was wrapped in a picnic blanket next to the canal, listening to Leonard Cohen croon "Suzanne" over and over. Leonard was nearby, leaning against one of the mature maples by the water's edge, his eyes hidden in the shadow of his signature fedora. He was singing to me. It was a cliché Cohen dream, but oh so lovely. The fantasy was cut short when another voice cut in. My mother.

"SUSAN! HELP!"

I jolted up from the mattress, pulled on an oversized T-shirt and stumbled into the hall, stopping short in the dining room doorway. My mother was lying face-up on the carpet. Nancy was kneeling over her, pinning our mother down with her thighs, arms crossed in defiance.

"What the fuck?" My voice croaked from cigarettes and too little sleep. "Get her off me!"

"You shouldn't have said that!" Nancy shouted at full throttle.

"Are you okay, Mom?" I asked, feeling useless.

"I'm not hurting her!" Nancy roared.

I wasn't convinced. Lately, my sister's outbursts had gained momentum—a shove, a plate thrown on the floor. She'd bit me once. None of these acts, however, had been unprovoked. I wondered what our mother had said.

"Tell her to get off!" My mother's voice was strained under Nancy's weight.

I grabbed Nancy's waist from behind and pulled, a useless manoeuvre. She turned and swatted my shoulder.

"Ouch!"

"This is *my* business, not yours."

I backed away, rubbing my shoulder. "Okay, okay, take it easy."

"I don't want to take it easy!"

"This is crazy, Nancy, listen to reason."

She glared at me. "I am *not* reasonable."

My sister's words were calculated, measured.

"Tell her we'll call the police," my mother said, her voice reduced to a whimper.

"I'll call the police myself!" Nancy yelled.

"Get off or I'll call Dad!" I yelled back, a last-ditch attempt.

Nancy rolled off our mother and pushed up from the floor, then disappeared down the hall to her bedroom. Our father was more of a threat than the police.

"What got her so mad?" I asked.

Our mother sat up and brushed invisible dust off her arms.

"She refused to get out of bed."

"Why not let her sleep?"

"That's not acceptable behaviour in this household."

Our mother's face was pasty white. The arguments drained her. They drained all of us, sucking out the precious little oxygen in the apartment. I wanted to live somewhere else, anywhere else than this airless fortress. Surely, my sister felt the same. Maybe everyone did.

"What time did you get home? Norman said it was light out."

If he knew, then why was she asking? I clucked my tongue, sighed loudly, and raised my hands to my hips, insolent gestures that, not long ago, would have resulted in punishment. My mother's beady eyes burned holes in my back as I headed for the bathroom. The heat in my chest stirred an allegiance with my sister, a feeling worth exploring, but I needed two Aspirin and I really had to pee.

A grey December 2019 sky shrouded Montreal in limbo. The parking lot beside Beaver Lake was a wasteland, waiting for the first snowfall and the winter enthusiasts laden with skates, skis and toboggans. I followed the footpath to the lookout at Mount Royal, a brisk, ten-minute walk. Visibility was poor; most of the city was enveloped in cloud, unlike the crisp atmosphere a few days earlier when I'd met Nancy at the food court and later drove Willy's friends to the abandoned factory. Directly below the lookout, the white stone pillars of the Port-Royal stood out like a beacon in the grey. I shuddered and turned away, surprised how the fortress still affected me after so many years.

Retracing my steps to Beaver Lake, I made a small detour through the gates at Mount Royal Cemetery. Seven Decembers earlier, I'd chosen a plot for my mother next to the road; my ailing father wouldn't have far to walk. He died three months later, before the ground had thawed. In the end, my parents' burial was synchronized, like so many aspects of their married life.

I approached the simple granite headstone and made a mental note to refrain from telling Nancy about my solo cemetery visit, which might trigger a "you went there without me" response. The English ivy covering the grave was still summer green; Lorna's endless energy was feeding the roots, even in December. Recently, I'd thrown away the weekly letters my mother had written from Germany and later from London, an action I now regret. In every letter, she had asked about Nancy and thanked me for watching over my sister. Surely, our mother had been haunted by guilt. The dementia may have been her final escape. I wept over the English ivy that would soon be covered by snow; seven years and the hole in my heart was far from healed.

11

I VACATED MY PARENTS' PORT-ROYAL APARTMENT while they were at
their Laurentian cottage for Labour Day weekend. The clandestine move
was cowardly, and the repercussions were bound to be severe; I was bail-
ing halfway through our twelve-month agreement. With no furniture or
furnishings, packing was easy; writing a note for my parents was less so.
Five crumpled drafts had been thrown in the trash. The final version left
on their kitchen counter was succinct—a phone number and five words:
"Will explain when you call."

Doug, an older friend in his late twenties, agreed to transport my belongings in his car to Libby's new home, a lower duplex in Notre-Dame-
de-Grâce. I'd had my fill of downtown stresses and looked forward to
a residential neighbourhood. Doug was a passionate Marxist-Leninist
who had taken part in the '68 riot in Concordia's computer room. He
took pleasure in helping me escape from the "capitalist fortress." Instead
of using the underground garage per Port-Royal protocol, he parked outside the main entrance with the motor running. We lugged five garbage
bags of clothes and three boxes of books from my parents' apartment
into the elevator and smiled at the disgruntled residents when the doors
opened on the fifteenth, tenth and fourth floors. Giovanni was standing
at attention in the lobby. The polished brass buttons of his crisp navy
jacket matched the handle of the door he held open. The faint twinkle
in his eyes, I hoped, was amusement and not relief to be rid of a scruffy
tenant in sweatpants and old sneakers. I flashed him my best smile and
passed through the glass door. A garbage bag caught on the concrete

step, tearing the thin plastic. Toiletries cascaded down the stairs to the sidewalk. Doug heaved the other four bags in his trunk along with the boxes and helped me gather up the spillage. We jumped in the car and Doug stepped hard on the gas, leaving behind a cloud of black smoke from his sputtering muffler.

The single piece of furniture in my new bedroom was a musty-smelling mattress left behind by the previous tenant. I sprayed the bed with Lysol and opened the window that overlooked our back deck. The room filled with a surf-like whoosh from the traffic on the nearby Décarie Expressway. The deck was massive, ideal for parties and sleeping under the stars on a warm night. Energized by possibility, I sorted my clothes into small piles, hung a beach towel across the window and stacked my books for a makeshift coffee table. I spread a blanket over the mattress and collapsed, drained from my little big move.

A ringing phone woke me. I rushed into the kitchen, disoriented and blinking. My hand wavered over the receiver before picking up.

"Hello?"

"This is Norman speaking."

I pulled my shoulders back and inhaled deeply. "Hi, Dad. Remember I mentioned how Libby was moving—"

He cut me off with a barrage of accusations—I was sneaky, dishonest, a liar, a slovenly slut. "You gave your word, Susan. A full year."

"I was afraid to—"

He cut me off a second time. I lacked integrity, could not be trusted, had let the family down.

My plan had been to apologize for being a coward and beg forgiveness. Instead, I gripped the phone and winced from the blows. Finally, they stopped. "This is about me, Dad. *My* needs."

"Narcissist," he muttered and hung up.

I stepped away from the phone, dizzy from my father's desperation. He needed me there to round out our crazy family. That wasn't love; that was possession. I wiped away my tears with the back of my hand.

"Have a seat," Libby said from the kitchen table. She was wearing a silky black bathrobe and her wild mane of russet hair was pinned up. Her pale face glowed under the pendulum kitchen lamp like a Jane Austen hero. Libby had her own issues with family. She knew crazy. We were both twenty-one, but she was light years ahead, a worldly soul who had lived in multiple cities. I often asked for her advice as I would an older sister, something I'd never done with my own. I slipped into the kitchen chair. She patted my shoulder and raised her cup of tea in salutation. I had made a clean break.

Nancy moved out of the Port Royal a few weeks after me, perhaps inspired by my escape. Her apartment near McGill University was a practical five-minute walk to her classes in the master's art education program. Our parents co-signed the lease without protest.

The glass door of the building was smeared with student fingerprints. The entranceway reeked of roach spray. I pressed the button below my sister's name and navigated across the faded tiles on the lobby floor that were littered with unopened junk mail. An Out of Order sign was taped to the elevator.

The studio apartment was furnished with family artifacts: ballerina bedspread; dresser with a missing bottom drawer handle; vintage school desk; our mother's Susie Cooper teapot. Nancy made us instant coffee with water boiled on a small gas stove next to a mini fridge. We sat at our parents' card table, unused since Etobicoke days. Nancy's foot tapped on the scratched parquet floor. Her hair had grown to the same length as the Hayley Mills days, but the strawberry hue had faded to dirty blond. The front of her navy blue sweater was stained with something white— toothpaste, maybe.

"Dad wants you to come for lunch on Saturday," she said.

I hadn't spoken to our parents for two months, not since my father's phone call when I'd moved in with Libby. A week ago, they'd moved to a smaller apartment one floor down, according to my sister.

"Will you be there?" I asked.

Nancy looked over at her desk. "I have to study."

Lucky her. I dreaded facing them alone.

Saturday, a few minutes before noon, the numbers on the panel flickered in quick succession like flash cards until they stopped at the eighteenth floor. I walked down the hallway towards my parents' door. We exchanged rushed kisses on the cheeks and they hurried me inside. Their apartment was a carbon copy of the one directly overhead, minus a bedroom and the housekeeping quarters. The furniture, however, was entirely new. The chintz sofa, my mother told me, had been purchased under the counsel of a designer who had also recommended the Murano glass chandelier, the art deco mirror and the coffee table with gold trim. I smiled and responded with words like "nice" and "lovely." The marked departure from my parents' simple style was unsettling.

My mother played the new Billy Joel CD they'd purchased in New York. I had no idea they'd been on a trip. The music, like the furniture, was not my taste but hip for a couple approaching their sixties. From my seat on the chintz sofa, I observed my father tapping his foot and swaying to the beat while my mother sang. She knew all the lyrics. Their performance was loose and relaxed. I didn't trust it. Something was up. My mother asked my father to play the song again. My father joined in this time. "Leave me alone." "This is my life." My new life without you. I felt a sharp jab.

Lunch was prepared and waiting on the table, a menu my parents would eat for years to come. The sardines were laid out in a fan over a bed of iceberg lettuce. The platter was rimmed with cherry tomatoes placed evenly apart, cut in half and sprinkled with salt. A stinky round cheese sat on a breadboard, next to that a plate of sliced cucumbers. And wine. Lots of wine.

Midway through the meal, my father studied my barely touched food.

"Sardines are good for you, full of iron," he said.

"I had a late breakfast."

Under his surveillance, I speared a tomato that I knew would taste like sardines. Everything on my plate tasted fishy. I chewed slowly and swallowed. He returned to his discussion with my mother: a corporate acquisition in Hamburg, Germany, that the president wanted him to oversee. A piece of tomato skin stuck to the back of my throat. I gagged, attracting my mother's eye. I reached for the water glass, then excused myself. My heart had started to thump wildly. I locked the bathroom door and curled up in a ball on the floor. The marble felt cool and steadying. My heart calmed. I reached for the counter and pulled myself up. My face looked pale in the mirror.

"Care for a slice?" my mother asked when I returned to the table. She pushed the smelly cheese towards me. I thought of telling her that I felt unwell. Maybe she would make it better like she did when I was a child. But she might also make it worse, a risk I didn't want to take.

I shook my head. "No thanks."

"How are your classes?" she asked.

"Not bad."

I had lied. University was competing with my evening shifts at the radio station. Unknown to my parents, I'd dropped a class. My father didn't approve of part-time anything. The younger daughter he'd been counting on was another fuck-up. The thumping in my chest returned. My legs were shaking. I carried my plate to the kitchen, declined dessert and thanked my parents, feigning a date with a study group at McGill. Another lie.

The fresh air on the sidewalk revived me. Suddenly, I was ravenous. I headed for the closest café, blaming my weak condition on low blood sugar; my diet was deplorable. The palpitations returned a week later in a crowded metro car. From that point forward, I avoided elevators, rode the bus instead of the metro and stayed clear of overbearing people, except family, of course. I had no clue that my condition was from anxiety and mild depression. With so much noise in our family, my quiet pain had slipped under the radar.

Three days following the grim visit to Mount Royal Cemetery, Nancy arrived at my front door in a terrible mood following an altercation with her painting instructor at Les Impatients, a non-profit like L'Atelier, with a mission to promote mental health through artistic expression. The instructor had directed too much attention on an attractive young female student and her boyfriend, multiple triggers for Nancy's insecurity. Worse still, the instructor didn't believe that once upon a time, Nancy had earned six credits towards a master's degree in art education, at least that was what Nancy said. I wondered if the art sessions at Les Impatients, less structured than L'Atelier, were a sad reminder of her past life in the studio, the impressive paintings, ceramics and lino prints she once produced and the art therapy career she never pursued. *Perhaps, I will eventually work with a wide cross-section of people who could benefit from therapy through art,* she wrote in her 1981 university application. Perhaps not. Nancy could still pick up a brush and paint a perfect contour of a face, a figure, a flower. But she usually stopped there. A few weeks later, Nancy would leave Les Impatients. She wanted to be the teacher, not the patient.

"Take a seat while I finish preparing lunch," I said.

Nancy flopped down on the kitchen bar stool next to the back door. "What are we eating?"

"I didn't have time to do anything fancy. I'm making salami and cheese sandwiches. All organic."

"I have salami at home."

I lathered the whole-grain bread with veggie mayo and Dijon and topped them with slices of Genoa and havarti. "Well, that's too bad 'cause it's all I got."

"You didn't go to much trouble."

I sighed. My knife dropped into the sink with a clang. "You don't have to eat the sandwich."

"I don't have much choice. I'm hungry."

She removed her wool sweater and fussed through her bag, waiting for me to finish preparing the food. The back door clicked shut; I had deliberately left it open a crack.

"I'm cold," Nancy said.

She was wearing a pale blue tank top.

"Why don't you put your sweater back on?"

Silence.

"Please open the door again. Just a crack."

"It's December."

"It's mild out. And you have a wool sweater hanging over the back of your stool."

"*It's mild out. You have a wool sweater,*" she said, imitating my voice.

My ears buzzed with a low hum, an engine starting up.

"It's my house," I muttered.

"Your house! I have a crappy apartment."

"You live in a rental condo with stainless steel appliances."

"This is not a very welcoming lunch."

"Please open the bloody door. A crack. Is that too much to ask?"

Nancy slapped her hands together, a thunderous clap two feet from my face. Years of experience warned me to walk away at this point. But the assault felt too personal, especially in my home sanctuary. She was not the only one who could fight. "If you continue to act like this, you'll have to leave this house."

She bellowed, a blood-curdling scream—"YOUR PERFECT HOUSE!"— then stood up, knocking over the bar stool as she grabbed the handle and pulled. The door banged against the dining room wall, leaving a dent I would later discover. She marched onto the back deck in her socks.

"Don't be an idiot," I cried. "The deck's sopping wet with melted snow."

I flopped the sandwiches on two plates and stepped over the overturned stool to the open door. She was standing with her back against the deck railing, arms folded, leering at me in a sinister sisterly way.

"I need a pair of dry socks and some water in a plastic cup."

"I have socks, but no plastic cup."

"I need PLASTIC."

I filled a paper coffee cup and handed it to her from the doorway. "I need you to leave now, Nancy."

She grabbed the cup and threw its contents at me. Whether it was deliberate or a sudden spasm from the medication was anyone's guess, although I'm pretty sure I knew which one it was. She shoved past me into the living room, sprawled lengthwise on the sofa and glared with a come-and-get-me expression. I moved in the opposite direction, to the far end of the kitchen, where I leaned face down on the counter and sobbed quietly, out of view. A minute later, I called my son.

"What's wrong?" Willy asked.

"Nancy's on one of her rampages," I whispered. "She refuses to leave."

"Then you leave. She won't stay without you."

"I don't wanna leave. This is my home. Can you come over? I need you."

Willy arrived ten minutes later.

"Why did you call him?" Nancy asked from the sofa.

"I needed help."

She shot up to sitting and grabbed the dry socks I'd left on the coffee table. Then she left. I slumped down on the bar stool and leaned over the counter, my face in my hands. Willy brought me one of the salami sandwiches. His hand stroked my back.

"Mom, why so sad? She's gone."

"Gone for how long? You know she'll be calling in an hour. I'm so sick of this. It's been going on too long."

I hated myself for whimpering in front of my son. I hated her. My heart pounded and my stomach turned. I pushed the plate away. There was no escape, not even in my home.

12

ON CHRISTMAS EVE AT THE DINNER TABLE, my new boyfriend, Jean-Pierre, a psychology student, told my parents and Nancy how he'd been raised in a working-class neighbourhood in the north end of Montreal. My father puckered his lip into a scowl. I was surprised that a self-made man from modest English roots had become a snob; only later would I understand that the feigned superiority was fed by a fear of slipping back. After the dishes were washed and put away, Nancy retired upstairs. Her evening meds made her drowsy. Jean-Pierre and I settled on the rattan sofa, a foot of distance between us. I'd warned him that holding hands would push the risk calculation into the red. In my final year at McGill, the finance professor taught us that risk is calculated by multiplying the probability of an event occurring with the consequences should that event occur. Risk equals likelihood times severity. Unsure about inviting Jean-Pierre for Christmas, I constructed a five-point scale grid and assigned the likelihood of my father losing his cool with my boyfriend five points and the severity of the consequences four points. The multiplied result pushed the risk far into the red zone. I invited him anyway.

A neighbour dropped by for a drink. My parents didn't socialize with cottage people, but this wealthy and recently divorced banker was an exception. He leaned back in the armchair, lifted his feet onto the ottoman and balanced a glass of Scotch on his belly. (If Jean-Pierre had done the same, my father would have cut his throat.) The banker oozed with confidence from a silver-spoon upbringing. I wondered if my father had invited him to intimidate the new boyfriend. The banker caught me staring and cocked his head, sizing me up. My parents had surely not told him I was living in Jean-Pierre's sketchy apartment under the Jacques Cartier Bridge, where the walls shook every time a truck drove across the span.

"I hear you recently graduated. What are you up to?" he asked me.

"Market research with a small consulting firm. You wouldn't know the name." I didn't mention it was a temporary job to make a bunch of money so I could fly to Europe.

"Impressive! What projects are you working on?"

"Nothing exciting. Foot cream."

"Tell me about the foot cream."

"I had to recruit seventy-five women for a product test."

"A-ha! A pilot study! How much did you pay them?"

"Sadly, I wasn't given a budget. It's a small firm."

"How the hell did you find seventy-five women then?"

"I accosted them in the lobby of our office building."

"How many did you get?"

"Three before the security guard chased me away."

The banker leaned back and roared. My father and Jean-Pierre frowned like they had when they heard the story a few weeks earlier. My mother, a little tipsy, was giggling.

"Then what?" he asked, wiping his eyes.

"I recruited the remaining seventy-two in the foot care aisle at Pharmaprix."

"You've got what it takes, girl," he said. "You'll be a member of the Mount Royal Club before long."

I'd been to the Mount Royal Club for lunch in honour of a scholarship sponsored by my father's company. The president and my father strode in through the front door while my mother, the president's secretary and I entered via the side entrance. The food was a great disappointment: organ meat. Sardines would have been better.

"When did they start letting women join the Mount Royal Club?" I asked, winking at my mother.

The neighbour took a long gulp from his glass.

"You won't give them a choice!" he replied.

My father beamed with approval. I had stepped into the game. I wished my boyfriend would do the same. The banker was friendly and funny. Instead, Jean-Pierre was drumming on the cover of a psychology textbook balanced on his lap. I reached for the Scotch. It was Christmas Eve, after all. We soon emptied the bottle and the banker said goodbye. My father locked the front door and returned to the living room. Jean-Pierre's textbook, now open on the coffee table, absorbed him.

"You didn't say much," my father said to him in a low voice that made me stiffen.

Jean-Pierre stood up from the sofa and stretched his arms over his head, oblivious to my father's accusatory tone.

"Your neighbour and I don't have much in common," he said, yawning.

My father blinked. He had been expecting something else, an apology or a grovel. His eyes sparkled like a rough sea. I wished to be anywhere else but that living room.

"You were quiet because you're envious."

Jean-Pierre guffawed. "Envious? That's ridiculous! I just didn't like the man."

"You didn't like our guest?" my mother piped in.

It was fruitless to point out that my boyfriend was also a guest. My father and Jean-Pierre's eyes had already locked, a clear indication that the risky event I'd been dreading had occurred and consequences were about to explode. My father's attitude may have changed had he heard Nancy's story that she later shared with me; the banker's brother once took advantage of her in the back seat of his car on a warm July evening while the banker and our parents partied in our living room, less than a hundred feet away. Not the banker's fault, of course. But was Jean-Pierre so evil?

"You didn't like our guest?" my father repeated. "What kind of idiot thing is that to say?"

Jean-Pierre was highly intelligent and didn't take kindly to being called otherwise. I braced myself for his rebuttal.

"You don't know how to love your daughters," he said quietly.

A nerve had been hit. My father's Scotch glass flew from his hand and crashed against the ceiling. He lunged forward with a fist of fury. Jean-Pierre, thirty-five years younger and sober, ducked to the side, his psychology textbook neatly tucked under his arm.

"Dad! Stop!" I shouted.

My father lowered his arm and glowered at me.

"Did you hear what he just said? How dare he blame me for Nancy's illness!"

"That's not what he said, Dad."

Jean-Pierre, in fact, had meant exactly that. He'd heard my family stories and concluded that Nancy's illness might have been avoided, or at least controlled, in a more accepting and loving family environment. But why couldn't he suck it up for my sake, for the sake of Christmas Eve? My father was right: my boyfriend was an idiot. They were both idiots. I glanced over at my mother, who was sweeping up the shattered glass and muttering to herself. No help there.

Nancy appeared in her pink-checkered flannel pajamas. Her eyes were puffy and half-closed.

"What's going on?" she asked, wavering side to side.

My father dismissed her.

"Nothing to see. Go to bed," he barked, an order a parent would give a small child. For a change, she wasn't in the spotlight. Nancy turned and went back upstairs. Jean-Pierre and I followed.

"We're leaving," Jean-Pierre growled in the upstairs hall.

Nine o'clock on Christmas Eve without a car, we were crazy to leave. But I remembered the risk grid: staying at the cottage would upgrade the severity of consequence from four points to five. Suicidal.

"Don't go," Nancy whispered. She'd been looking forward to sharing her room with me. Sleeping with a boyfriend at our parents' cottage, even in our twenties, was strictly taboo.

"They gave me no choice, Nance. Sorry."

"You have all the luck. You can leave."

I didn't feel lucky. Armoured with ski jackets, toques, mittens and winter boots, Jean-Pierre and I lugged our bags up the steep driveway. My parents shouted accusations from the open front door. I stopped to catch my breath, my heart pounding with emotion. Nancy's silhouette glowed from her bedroom window.

Jean-Pierre nudged me. "Come on. Let's go!"

No shining stars to guide us along the five-kilometre dirt road. We walked in the dark for twenty minutes before a car picked us up. Two rides later, we staggered through Jean-Pierre's front door.

"Your dad wants you to marry a successful businessman," he murmured from under the sheets. I wiggled away to the far edge of the mattress, angry at my boyfriend's behaviour, my father's aggression, my mother's diehard allegiance to her husband and my sister's illness that redirected parental attention to me. The metal bed frame started to vibrate, a heavy truck crossing the bridge, the fifth in the past hour. Ten more would pass over before the low rumbling finally put me to sleep.

Christmas 2019 arrived in the city. Dinner had been prepared and was keeping warm in the oven. Candles flickered from the dining room table set for nine. Six adult children were scattered over the living room—two were mine, and two were Keith's, plus their partners. They took turns nibbling at the cheese and fruit platters on the coffee table. The Tragically Hip was playing in the background. A tidy pile of presents from Secret Santa lay under the Christmas tree at the far end of the room, one present per person to avoid mass spending. I sank into the sofa, sandwiched between my son and daughter, and winked at my husband across from me. A perfect moment.

Boots stamped on the front porch and a key struggled in the lock. I brushed the cracker crumbs off my lap and headed for the front door.

"The lock's broken," Nancy said, pushing past me.

I inhaled deeply, barely recovered from her outburst a few weeks earlier when she'd upturned a chair, doused me with water and refused to move from the sofa.

"The lock works fine," I told her. "You need to pull the door towards you before turning the key."

"It's broken. You should replace it."

The argument could have started there, but I let it go. Christmas.

Armed with a shopping bag full of presents, she stepped off the doormat in full winter gear and marched down the hallway to the living room, leaving a trail of melted slush on the hardwood floor. The argument could have started there, but I ran to the kitchen in search of paper towels. Christmas.

"Ho ho ho! Gifts for everyone!" my sister shouted.

She handed her bag to Willy, who placed the presents under the tree. Nancy had ignored my repeated reminders of Secret Santa. The argument could have started there, but instead, I bent down on hands and knees to clean the floor. Christmas.

"Can you take this?" Nancy asked, handing her coat to Keith.

"Don't forget your boots," he said.

She looked down at the floor and frowned as if noticing her messy trail for the first time.

"Pass me the paper towels. I can clean that," she told me.

"It's okay, I'm almost done."

She bent down and grabbed the roll. "My boots wouldn't be so wet if someone had driven me here," she muttered.

"I was busy with the meal, and it's only a ten-minute bus ride."

"A bus ride on Christmas?"

"At least you don't have to cook for nine people," I said.

The argument could have started there, but Sarah called out from the sofa. "Nancy, come in and join us!" Christmas.

Nancy crossed her arms and studied the spot where I'd been sitting.

"There's no room for me there."

Sarah bolted to standing. "Then take my seat."

"Thank you, but I'd rather stand for now."

My sister grabbed a gift from under the tree. Sarah looked over and winked. She knew the drill. Secret Santa would have to wait. Like every Christmas, Nancy was struggling for control, a holiday tradition. My children were accustomed to her need for attention, especially on family occasions.

"Can someone turn off that wailing?" Nancy asked, pointing at the stereo.

"I'm going to check on the turkey," I said on my way to the kitchen. The only thing that needed checking was the rage burning within me. The Tragically Hip was replaced by my sister's stage whispers, the two S's in my name. I pictured her posed in the middle of the living room, firing multiple complaints about me to my loved ones. Keith and the kids wouldn't take her seriously, but my mind was blurred by resentment. If I were that evil, then why would I invite her year after year? I charged out of the kitchen, my rage unleashed. Regret would come later.

13

SUMMER OF 1980, MY FATHER WAS IN SANTIAGO negotiating a lumber agreement with General Pinochet's Chilean government when my fifty-eight-year-old mother called about sharp pains in her chest. My grand-mother, whom I'd never met, had died at fifty-seven from a massive stroke. My mother refused to call an ambulance. The pain wasn't bad enough, she said. The Montreal General Hospital was in plain view of her Port-Royal living room window. She could walk. Finally, we agreed; she would allow Giovanni to call a taxi. I would meet her at the emergency.

The triage nurse led me to a curtained-off room.

"You were quick," my mother said.

Her smile was weak, but her eyes were alert. She was staring down at my left hand, which I quickly hid behind my back. The nurse wheeled an electrocardiograph into the curtained-off room, saving me from giving my mother an explanation. I hoped she would forget what she'd seen.

"Normal," the nurse said, removing the electrodes. "Likely not a heart attack, but your blood pressure is a little high. We'll know more from the blood work."

My mother turned to me.

"Do you have something to tell me?" she asked, her eyebrows arching.

In a panic, I had forgotten to remove the engagement ring that I'd been hiding during parental visits.

"It's a ring, nothing more," I answered.

"Good. Twenty-three is far too young for marriage."

I agreed but wasn't about to let her know that.

The doctor diagnosed my mother with coronary artery disease, and she was moved to the cardiac ward for a ten-day stay. In between jobs, I was happy to step into the role of bedside companion. Following a three-month European adventure, Jean-Pierre and I had recently moved to a third-floor walk-up in the Plateau-Mont-Royal, four blocks from Leonard Cohen's house. My parents and I were still estranged following the Jean-Pierre Christmas blowout six months earlier. They were also displeased by my unemployment and living situation. Helping my mother in the hospital was an opportunity for redemption and reconnection. On day two of sitting vigil, my father returned from Chile. He was grateful for my presence given his extreme dislike of hospitals. My mother shooed him away after ten minutes and squeezed my hand, telling me I was a model hospital visitor. Nancy's presence was as brief as our father's; a dark and handsome engineering student named Husain was distracting her. The ten days passed quickly. My eyes were misty on the morning of my mother's discharge, as if I was saying goodbye.

Six months later, slamming sticks from a street hockey game woke me. I stretched and listened for sounds of life in the apartment. Nothing. Jean-Pierre had already left for the university library. We rarely saw each other since I'd started my new job with a marketing firm. This was my first Saturday off in eight weeks. A morning to myself! I scuttled across the cold bedroom floor and raised the blind. Fresh snow clung to the window screen. Below, the street was a powdery blur.

The telephone rang while I was making coffee.

"I'm in trouble," my sister said.

I dropped two tablespoons of coffee beans into the grinder.

"What's up?" I asked.

"I took some Tylenol."

"Hold on," I pressed on the grinder and counted to ten. "What was that about Tylenol?"

"I took too many."

I patted the coffee grounds into the stovetop espresso maker and turned the gas on high. "How many is too many?"

"Half a bottle."

I asked the taxi driver to hurry. It was an emergency. To save time, he drove the wrong way down my sister's street and braked in front of her building. I scrambled up the steps, two at a time. Nancy had recently moved one block east into another cruddy apartment close to the university. I found her on the lobby floor, crouched against a wall.

"Nance!" I cried, rushing to her.

She looked up and smiled, a goofy grin. Relieved, I grinned too.

The taxi dropped us off at the Montreal General Hospital. The emergency room was packed. Nancy was lucid, able to walk, but the mention of "overdose" rushed us to triage.

"Are you going to call Mom and Dad?" she asked, pushing up from the narrow bed.

I shook my head. Our parents were at the cottage, an hour and a half away. Nancy closed her eyes. Two minutes later, she was snoring. I made a break for the coffee dispenser in the lobby, the world's worst brew.

A young psychiatrist with deep blue eyes and dark hair that curled around a cherubic face explained that my sister hadn't taken enough pills to be in danger. Perhaps it was a cry for attention? Regardless, she needed to undergo a psychological evaluation, as per hospital protocol.

"Do you have suicidal thoughts?" he asked my sister.

She was eyeing him, suddenly wide awake.

"You must be a student," she said.

His cheeks flushed. "I'm a resident."

"My boyfriend is a resident. Do you have a girlfriend?"

"What's his name, this resident?" asked the young psychiatrist, avoiding her question. "Maybe I know him."

I interjected. "He lives in a university residence. Not quite the same as a resident."

"Potato, tomato," Nancy replied.

I was used to my sister's jumbled expressions and knew what she meant. Judging from the puzzled look on the young psychiatrist's face, he did not. I sat back in the chair and unbuttoned my jacket. The evaluation would be a lengthy one. My sister's cry for attention was working.

Forty-five minutes later, we were dismissed. I peeked at the open file on the desk. "Low risk for suicide." Nancy chuckled when I told her. "Duh," she said. I was too relieved to be angry. We left the hospital and walked down Côte-des-Neiges and turned east on Sherbrooke. The snow had stopped falling and the sky was a brilliant blue. Nancy waved at a panhandler positioned in front of the Musée des beaux-arts, his gloved hand open for offerings.

"Hi!" she shouted.

The panhandler turned and flashed Nancy a smile.

"You know him?" I asked.

"I know lots of people downtown. This is where I live, remember?"

We turned south on rue de la Montagne. Nancy stopped in front of the Coffee Mill and offered to buy me anything I wanted. She was in an upbeat mood. Hanging out for a bit was a good idea, something we rarely did.

"I have a confession," she said between sips of cappuccino.

"Go for it."

She described how a group of Hare Krishna dancers had approached her when she was watching their performance down the street, in front of Ogilvy's huge glass window. They had invited her to join them for a movie and cake at their headquarters somewhere north of the city, she wasn't sure where.

"Are you nuts?" I asked, shocked. Hare Krishna was a more serious threat to my sister than a minor Tylenol overdose.

She waved her hand. "Perfectly safe. I wasn't alone."

"What happened?"

"First, we watched the movie."

"What kind of movie?"

"No idea. The volume was cranked too high. I covered my ears."

"Then what, after the movie?"

"We sat in a circle and introduced ourselves. When it was my turn, I stood up and started singing and dancing, just like I've seen them do on the street corner. They looked at each other, you know how people do. I didn't like that at all. I told them I had a mental illness and didn't like being stigmatized."

"Did they apologize?"

"They asked me to leave."

"Did you?"

"I insisted on eating the cake they'd promised."

Coffee spurted out of my mouth over the table, which made me laugh even louder. My fear was unfounded. My sister didn't take kindly to orders from cults or otherwise. She picked up the bill, and we spent the next couple of hours wandering east along Ste-Catherine. Free of family, hospital and possibly some of her medication, my sister had become familiar with every store, every restaurant, every church and every panhandler. Those downtown years were the best of her life, she told me years later.

The phone rang for the third time in the past hour. I didn't feel like talking to my sister after the Christmas blowout three days earlier. I had been controlling myself for the sake of the blended family, but then I had exploded. I couldn't remember eating the turkey dinner we'd worked so hard to prepare. I was still upset with her and myself, my lack of control. Keith assured me it didn't matter. But we all knew better. I glanced over at the ringing phone and blinked. It wasn't Nancy; it was an "unknown caller," which could mean the hospital or the police.

"Hello?"

"Is this Nancy's sister?"

"Yes."

"My name is Marie. I'm calling from Tel-Aide Québec."

Tel-Aide is a listening service for people experiencing emotional distress.

"Is my sister okay?"

"We're concerned. She says she can't get a hold of you and wants to kill herself. She gave us your number."

I rolled my eyes.

"Are you there?" Marie asked.

"Yes, still here."

"She gave us your number."

"Of course she did."

"Your sister was very descriptive, talked about stabbing herself with a kitchen knife, one she'd inherited from your mother."

Let her do it, I thought.

"She's low-risk, not suicidal," I said quietly.

"We can't take a chance, especially during holiday season. I would like to put her through to you. She's waiting on another line."

"Thank you, but I really don't need to speak with her."

"She says she must talk to you."

I felt bad for the Tel-Aide operator. She was just doing her job.

"Okay, put her through."

"Hello?" Nancy's voice was bright, cheery.

"Clever way to get through to me," I replied.

"I was worried when you didn't answer."

"Worried about me or worried about you?"

She grunted. "Why would I worry about you? You have a beautiful life."

I kept my lips tightly closed, refusing to fall into the trap.

"I hung out with the homeless man yesterday, the guy who lives in Benny Park. He asked where I live."

"You didn't tell him, I hope. He could stalk you."

"Don't tell me that. I feel nervous enough."

"Nervous enough to plunge a knife in your heart?"

"Oh, that."

"That poor woman—Marie. She believed you."

"You're giving me shit again."

"You didn't give him your number, did you?"

"Who?"

"The homeless guy!"

"Course not, but I told him where I live."

"You did what?!"

"You're not my mother."

"Honestly, Nancy, I just want a quiet night by myself."

"Where's Keith?"

"He's at the cottage."

"Do you think I'm like Uncle Harry?" she asked.

Uncle Harry from Manchester pushed the stroller down the stairs. It sounded like an old English nursery rhyme. Our father, the baby in the family, had been in the stroller at the time. Years later, he signed the papers for Harry's lobotomy, a surgical procedure that severed his brother's prefrontal lobe, an attempt to make him normal. Harry lived the rest of his life in a group home, estranged from family.

"No, Nancy, You're not like Uncle Harry."

"Why didn't you answer before?"

"I was busy."

"Guess your life is more important than mine."

"Maybe it is," I replied coolly.

My eyes narrowed and the kitchen blurred. My fingers tightened on the phone that I wanted to smash against the granite counter. Instead, I grabbed a magazine and threw it at the dining room table, knocking over an empty vase. The day before, I'd engaged in a lengthy conversation about my sister with an old friend who called me a saint. A saint never resorts to violence.

I counted the seconds waiting for her to recite the next line. *One sister steamboat, two sister steamboat—*

"You're lucky you don't have a mental illness." Her fingers tapped against the mouthpiece.

My eyes started to water. A saint does not feel sorry for herself.

"I don't feel very lucky."

On the windowsill above the sink was a china bird that had belonged to my mother. It was missing a wing. Like the other broken and chipped items I've inherited, I couldn't bring myself to throw it out.

"Of course, you're lucky. Two husbands, two children, two houses—"

I hung up, switched the ringer to silent and tossed the phone. It slid off the counter onto the kitchen floor and started to vibrate with an incoming call. I sat down next to the phone. The floor was littered with food crumbs and the cupboard doors were streaked with fingerprints. My house would be immaculate if not for the non-stop demands and complaints, the multiple calls. I imagined her quavering soprano voice, blaming me for her lousy life. The undeserved accusation gripped my throat; it squeezed the life out of me. I curled into a ball and moaned like a crazy person, sick like my sister and cursed by our deceased parents. Thankfully, I was alone, no one to see me in this wacky state. How many times had I told Keith and the kids that I'm done? They stopped believing me ages ago.

14

MY SISTER WAS STATIONED INSIDE the glass-walled security booth at the university library. Her navy blazer, white button-down shirt and pulled-back hair made her appear older than twenty-nine. She looked up from her book and smiled at me, then straightened her mouth and lifted her eyebrows, all business and no play. I passed over my bag for a meticulous search that felt more like a sister inspection than a security check. She waved me forward into the library with a poker face even when I saluted her and stuck out my tongue. I zipped up my bag, turned my back on the turnstiles and headed for the street, satisfied with my own sister inspection. Since the beginning of the semester, our parents had been concerned that Nancy was overextending herself with part-time work on top of three courses in the art education master's program. They had nothing to worry about—she was alert, on the job.

Nineteen eighty-three was a busy year for me as well. I had accepted a marketing position at Ernst & Young, moved into a street-level apartment on St. Denis, broken up with Jean-Pierre and fallen in love with Phil, who grew up five houses away from our former family home. I ignored my mother's comment: "You like Phil because he comes from a Westmount family with good credentials." She didn't understand the complexity of my ongoing struggle to belong since we'd left Toronto suburbia fifteen years earlier. Phil was descended from a well-established Anglo-Quebec lineage with strong roots in Montreal's Golden Square Mile, but he shared my distrust of mainstream convention and values—the perfect rebel partner for me! My sister had long given up on finding her way to fit in—to Quebec society or otherwise.

In the weeks following my impromptu library visit, we seldom heard from Nancy and when we did, the calls were brief and rushed. Unknown to us, she was easing off the medication that had been making her too sluggish to handle a full schedule. Off the pills, she became infused with an energetic high; it was impossible for her to remain still. We had no idea she was skipping class and missing work, the exact opposite of what she had intended. A week passed without any news; she didn't answer the phone or the apartment buzzer. My father reached out to the hospitals. He found Nancy on his second call. She had been admitted to the psychiatric ward, 4East, at the Montreal General Hospital following a 9-1-1 report that a young woman had been seen dancing on a rooftop. Apparently, Nancy had taken to eating and sleeping up there. The open sky liberated her from the confines of her apartment on the fifth floor. Up on the roof.

As the weeks passed, the possibility of a short hospital stay looked unlikely. My mother enlisted my help to clear Nancy's apartment. I was happy to oblige, a concrete way to help. The elevator arrived on the fifth floor of her building with a sudden jerk. The doors opened and the stacked pile of empty packing boxes spilled out. My mother and I carried what we could and kicked the other boxes down the hall. The janitor was jingling his keys, waiting in front of my sister's door. He let us in, peeked inside, then retreated, leaving us alone.

The apartment had been left in illogical disarray: clothes hanging in the kitchen, dishes stacked against the bedroom wall, a towel draped over the small television. The kitchen smelled like burning rubber, my sister's manic energy. My mother opened the windows despite the April rain. We worked in silence. She packed clothes and linen; I emptied rotting food from the fridge. A cookie sheet on a rack in the oven held a dozen round-shaped dark objects. I leaned in and braved a sniff. Mud cakes, my sister later explained, one of her cooking experiments. The kitchen counter was cluttered with condiments and spices for meals not yet prepared. On hands and knees, I pulled out a plastic bag wedged in the back of the cupboard under the kitchen sink. I shrieked at the contents: my thirteen-year-old sister's strawberry-blond hair.

"What's wrong?" my mother called out from the bedroom.

"Cockroach!" I lied.

My sister's dead hair would freak out my mother. I threw the plastic bag straight into the garbage, anxious to vacate my sister's former apartment.

After a two-month hospitalization that ended in late June, Nancy was transferred to a downtown halfway house on avenue du Musée. She made friends with a subdued Franco-Albertan named Justin who was staying in the room across the hall. Justin was a couple of years younger than Nancy, with brown shoulder-length hair and downward-looking eyes. He often wore loose-fitting Indian cotton shirts. Justin and Nancy soon became a couple. They moved out of the halfway house into their own apartment in Notre-Dame-de-Grâce, a few blocks west from where I used to live with Libby. Despite his slight frame, Justin carried a mattress on his back from the Salvation Army to their new home ten blocks away. Nancy was impressed. From outside appearances, she was settling down, playing house. Meanwhile, Justin's hair grew longer. He was looking more and more like Jesus in Leonardo de Vinci's *The Last Supper*. My parents and I never got to know him very well. The only sound he made in our presence was from the constant clinking of a metal spoon inside his coffee mug. Despite Justin's monastic silence and obsessive stirring, I was happy for my sister. She deserved love.

The honeymoon lasted three months.

Nancy called my parents in a fury. She told them that Justin had no money to pay the rent and that Justin had attacked her with a broom handle. He'd vanished by the time our furious parents turned up, never to be seen again. Distraught and fragile, Nancy spiralled into depression and was readmitted to 4East. Months passed and another apartment was emptied, this time with help from Phil, who had recently moved in with me. An indoctrination to the family, I told him as we lifted my sister's boxes into the rental truck. Meanwhile, Nancy was not responding to medication and the psychiatrist on 4East had requested a family meeting.

I sat beside my parents at a rectangular conference table. The wooden surface was worn and badly in need of varnish. My mother balanced a writing pad on her lap and was searching her purse for a pen. My father was staring out the window, perhaps looking for his office tower in the downtown skyline. He turned when the 4East staff entered the room: the occupational therapist, the physiotherapist, the social worker and the head nurse. They nodded and sat down across from us, shuffling papers in their files. Finally, the psychiatrist arrived and settled at the head of the table. In a suit and tie, he looked more like a lawyer than a doctor. He cleared his throat before speaking.

"Unfortunately, your daughter's condition appears to be chronic."

The 4East staff nodded in agreement. My parents looked confused.

"What exactly are you saying?" asked my mother, sharpness in her voice.

"We can't keep her here long-term. Our recommendation is a transfer to the Douglas Hospital. She will be better off in an environment that can provide appropriate care."

My father's head bowed. The pen in my mother's hand froze mid-air. I crossed my arms and squeezed my chest. Appropriate care? The Douglas was an insane asylum, a bughouse, a loony bin. Nancy was young, barely thirty. Why wouldn't they let her stay on 4East a little longer? The staff was silent. I wondered what they were thinking. Did they agree with the doctor? I prayed my parents would protest.

"If that is what you recommend, I suppose we have no choice," my father said in a low voice. The doctor made a note in the file. My mother returned the pen and pad to her purse and folded her hands on her lap. Her eyes were welling up. I could hear the dull roar of traffic on Cedar through the crack in the open window. Four stories down, in the parking lot, two women were laughing. I clenched my jaw at the injustice, my innocent sister sentenced to life imprisonment. The psychiatrist excused himself and the 4East staff dribbled out one by one. We were alone. My father was staring out the window again. My mother started to sob. I opened my bag and searched for gum or candy. Anything.

Nancy was waiting outside the conference room, slumped over in a plastic chair. Her face lit up when she saw us. She pushed up to standing, a hand on the wall for support. Our parents steered her down the hall and into her room, their arms crooked into hers. I waited in the doorway while our father broke the bad news. Nancy's slouch straightened with his words.

"It's for the best," said my father in a soft, tender voice that made me feel even worse. "They have specialists. Better doctors than here."

My sister freed herself from our parents' hold, crawled onto the bed and rolled onto her side, her back to us. I looked on, helpless. My parents were in charge. At twenty-six, I was still a child in this scenario.

Two months following my sister's transfer to the Douglas Hospital, a promising young upstart was promoted to a position that eliminated our father's job. As compensation, our father was offered a director post in a subsidiary operation in Hamburg, an acquisition he had helped orchestrate. I urged him to negotiate an early retirement package instead. He scoffed at the idea. Sixty-one, he said, was too young to retire. I suspected a deeper reason. The transfer to Germany would provide an exit strategy, a second chance. *Leave us alone, this is our life. Our new life without you.*

Birds abandon their young when one of them falls from the nest. The energy required to heal the injured baby bird threatens the survival of the nest, mother and father included. Nancy had fallen hard. Sixteen years battling with her illness had left my parents drained. Our mother promised to write us often. Our father said they would return for Christmas and the summer holidays. In the weeks leading up to their departure, meetings were arranged with the lawyer, the accountant and the investment advisor. I signed a power of attorney at the bank and a slew of other documents to act on my father's behalf during his absence. My parents' trust filled me with purpose. I was an adult. Responsible. They could count on me.

On a miserably cold New Year's Eve, I snuggled into the living room sofa and raised my wine to Keith.

"Here's to surviving another fucking Christmas."

"Come on," he said, clinking my glass. "It wasn't that bad."

He patted my shoulder, which made me feel even worse. My Grinch attitude towards the holidays was undeserving of sympathy.

"I wish we still had Casa Verano. We could celebrate the holiday far away from you-know-who."

"Come on," Keith said. "We always came home for Christmas. You insisted."

He was right, of course. I reached for my journal and pen. "Okay, time for 2020 resolutions."

Keith groaned. "You know I don't do that sort of thing."

I wagged my pen at him. "There must be at least one thing you want to change."

"Honestly, no. But you go ahead and make your own list."

The compulsion for resolutions stemmed from the paternal side of my family, a conclusion I'd made after discovering lists written by my father in a folder marked "personal." His resolutions weren't exclusively recorded on New Year's Eve; they were dated throughout the year. *February 3: Practice piano daily. June 26: Pursue a more rigorous exercise program. October 19: Find better ways to deal with stress.* I tapped the pen against my journal in a steady heartbeat rhythm while the unthinkable floated in my head. *December 31, 2019: Walk away from your sister.* I calculated my parents' age when they'd set up their new life in Hamburg. The result struck me with the force of a ten-foot wave. They were two years younger than I was now. The time was long overdue to leave the nest that I'd stepped back into thirty-five years ago, a nest that was not of my own making. The resolution sounded perfectly reasonable. Yet still, my pen wavered. Abandoning my sister felt akin to murder.

"What did you write?" Keith asked, peering over my shoulder.

I drained the glass in a long, final gulp.

"Find better ways to deal with stress."

He nodded with approval, perhaps as my mother had done when she'd read her husband's list. I curled into the sofa, enveloped by the warmth of the wine.

15

A COLONY OF SQUAWKING GULLS lifted off the spring grass and took flight over the narrow private road leading to the Douglas Hospital in Verdun, a southwestern borough of Montreal. I eased off the accelerator and lowered the window. A week earlier, the lilacs had started to bud. Now, the bushes were heady with sweet perfume. Eleven o'clock on a weekday morning, the visitor parking lot was almost empty. I steered into my usual spot facing the river on the other side of boulevard La-Salle. Sparkles of light danced over the rapids, beckoning me to the foot-path I had never used in the seven years that my sister had been in the Douglas. Her life was on ice; mine was mushrooming. Meditative walks along the St. Lawrence River did not fit into my crammed schedule. Five client files waited for me in my home office; I hoped to add a sixth as a result of a meeting that afternoon. Managing a small business wasn't the only change in my life. Despite our resistance to convention, Phil and I were married. A notary had presided over a two-minute ceremony on the lawn of Bar Harbor's Sea Coast Mission. After signing the no-tarial papers, we clambered over slippery rocks in our rubber boots and crouched on a ledge with a bottle of champagne and two glasses we'd taken from our motel bathroom. When my father heard the breaking nuptial news, he was convinced our American marriage in the State of Maine was invalid in Canada. Wishful thinking on his part; he didn't think highly of Phil.

I stepped out of the car, opened the trunk and reached for the empty suitcase my sister had requested. A muscle spasm in my lower abdomen drew back my hand. I was at the beginning of the third trimester, according to the ultrasound. My belly was hard and drawn tight like a drum, in expansion mode like the rest of my life, although the pregnancy still didn't show very much. The genetic counsellor at the Montreal Children's Hospital assured me that the likelihood of my baby developing schizophrenia later in life was one in a hundred, the same probability as the general population. My odds, as a direct sibling in the same generation, were much higher, closer to one in ten, she had said. I'd left the genetic counselling clinic with a buzzing head. Thirty-three was past the age of probable onset, but what if I wasn't typical? I swept the thought into a remote file at the back of my brain where I kept other unsettling questions. My fully booked schedule allowed no time for anxious speculation.

My sister was on the second floor of the Perry Pavilion, one of thirty-seven buildings on the 110-acre hospital property. A modern red brick entrance had been added to the nineteenth-century grey stone facade. I wheeled the empty suitcase towards a burly, bearded man in a black toque, navy plaid jacket and jeans who was standing next to the main door. I recognized him from previous visits. Running late, I rushed past him into the building.

"*Excusez-moi!*"

The solid tenor voice stopped me in my tracks. I turned. The man had followed me inside. I'd never heard him speak before.

"There's an elevator down the hall, Miss."

He spoke with a thick Québécois accent. I wondered why he was staying at an English psychiatric hospital instead of the French equivalent, Hôpital Louis-H. Lafontaine, on the opposite end of the Island of Montreal, twenty-two kilometres upstream. Nineteenth-century urban planners had made sure to keep the insane at a safe distance from the city core.

"*Merci*," I replied. "I prefer the stairs. *Les escaliers.*"

I shivered from my recent experience in an antiquated lift that had carried me at a halting gait to my parents' London flat, their new headquarters abroad since our father had retired. They had let go of their apartment in the Port-Royal; the Laurentian cottage was now their Canadian base from late spring until fall. For the duration of my London visit, I'd insisted on walking up and down the five flights of stairs. The physical exertion combined with my parents' endless walks and pauper diet led to a small weight loss, a phenomenon that concerned my obstetrician. (I regained the pounds in one week.) Apart from my brief London visit, our parents' new regime made little difference to my life. They still lived at arms-length from Nancy and me.

The burly, bearded man stepped closer and grinned. The coils in his facial hair looked complicated. His dark eyes were studying me. I wondered how he'd used his tenor voice in the past. Opera singer? Radio announcer?

"A-ha!" he cried. "You are claustraphobique."

Or maybe he'd been a psychologist. I gave him a thumbs-up followed by a friendly wave. In the outside world, I would have denied my phobia. Here, I fit right in. The wheels of the suitcase knocked against each stair, announcing my arrival to the second floor of the Perry Pavilion. I pressed the buzzer and stepped back. The staff on Perry 2C were overloaded; five minutes would often pass before someone unlocked the door. In her first few months at the Douglas, Nancy had stayed in an open ward with full privileges, like the burly, bearded man. She explored the hospital grounds and the labyrinth of underground tunnels, and then she ventured farther into the streets of Verdun. In the middle of a January freeze, a hospital employee found her in a snowbank outside the main gate without a coat. Shortly afterwards, she was moved to Perry 2C, a locked ward.

The door finally opened. One of the nurses, Mr. Malik, poked his head into the hallway with an affectionate smirk.

"Good morning, Ms. Grundy. I see from the suitcase that you're checking in."

I laughed. "Not quite yet, Mr. Malik."

"So, what's with the suitcase?"

"Nancy wants me to take some of her clothes."

He clicked his heels and snapped a salute. "Duty calls!"

He then turned, distracted by a prolonged howl behind him, possibly from the new patient, Patrick, whose room was at the far end of the hall. Then again, the howl could belong to anyone, including Nancy. My main take-away as a seven-year veteran visitor was that a locked ward was often a noisy ward. How did the staff manage? Were they self-medicated?

"Quick, come in before someone escapes," said Mr. Malik, winking.

"How's Nancy today?" I asked, grateful that the howling had ceased.

"A bad day, I'm afraid. You may end up talking to yourself."

Nancy had good days, bad days and ugly days. On good days, she would be dressed, showered and pacing the hall, waiting for my arrival. She would tell me about the other patients and read the latest letter from our mother, and I would read her mine. On "really" good days, she would be granted a two-hour pass. We would drive to McDonald's in LaSalle or walk over to a nearby depanneur in Verdun, where the owner never smiled despite the profit he made from selling cigarettes and snack food to his Douglas Hospital clientele. On bad days, I would find her sitting in a corner, skimpily dressed, no shoes, hair unwashed, no expression even when she recognized me—zombie sister. I never saw Nancy on ugly days. She was either heavily sedated or restrained in the "side room," a closet-size space with a small glass window facing the nursing station. According to Nancy, the lingering stench of urine and feces, too strong to be removed by ammonia, was as severe a punishment as the restraining jacket she was forced to wear.

I wheeled down the hall and turned into my sister's room. Expectations were low.

"Hi, Nance," I said softly.

She was lying face up on the bed. Her right eye opened a crack. A glimmer of light.

"I brought the suitcase you wanted."

No response. I moved in for a closer look. A sibling didn't have the same authority as a parent or partner to drill doctors with questions, at least that was how I felt in those days. Instead, I relied on my own observations and feedback from Mr. Malik. No drooling and her eyes weren't rolling upwards; she hadn't been sedated. The bad day was a result of a mood slump, not aggressive behaviour. A stack of neatly folded clothes was piled on the dresser that separated her bed from her roommate's. I removed the clothes and left half a dozen lemons in their place. The fruit shone like yellow stars in the dimly lit room. Nancy's right eye was still open a crack, but the light had dulled, and her breathing was heavy. I bent over to whisper goodbye. Her cheek smelled like roses. She'd managed a shower even on a bad day.

My exit coincided with the distribution of lunchtime meds. I wheeled the suitcase around the zigzag line of patients. Richard, a long-term resident like my sister, stepped out of the queue to greet me. His wide-open eyes were attached to an old man's body.

"Did you bring me a lemon like you promised?" he asked.

Richard and Nancy shared a passion for the sour fruit. I reached into my pocket and handed him one. He beamed in response. Ten years later, he would die, middle-aged, as would several other Perry 2C residents.

"Can I have a kiss?"

His watery green eyes reminded me of the Frog Prince. Offering him my cheek and allowing a quick peck would be a small sacrifice, but the corners of his mouth were caked with white spittle. I pulled away.

"Remember, Richard? We're saving the kiss for your birthday."

He stared at me blankly. I seized the opportunity to push on.

"My birthday is in three months and twenty days," he shouted.

I turned and smiled. "You'll have to remind me."

Richard clapped his hands, a child's response. Mr. Malik unlocked the steel door with one of the keys dangling from his belt and I descended to the main floor, puffing from the awkwardness of navigating a suitcase on stairs. Coming down was much harder than going up. Thankfully, Nancy's clothes weighed next to nothing, no strain on my abdomen. The burly, bearded man rushed to open the door and wished me a good day, the gatekeeper of the Perry Pavilion.

The following week, my sister's psychiatrist issued an overnight pass, a first for Nancy and me. Mr. Malik had reported five consecutive good days. Unheard of! She was waiting at the nursing station, her spring jacket zipped up and a bag on her arm.

"Good luck," said Mr. Malik, unlocking the door.

Under the shelter of an umbrella, I guided Nancy to the car and helped her settle in the passenger seat. The rain eased up as we pulled out of the parking lot. The narrow road was sprinkled with lilac blossom confetti.

"It feels like a wedding!" I cried.

Nancy smiled. "Speaking of weddings, Patrick and I did it in the storage closet this week."

I glanced at her sideways. "What do you mean by 'did it'?"

"We had sex."

"Did you use protection?"

"I don't need that anymore."

During the summer, a benign cyst had been removed from my sister's ovary. The surgeon suggested he perform a tubal ligation at the same time. Nancy consented, the practical thing to do, she said.

"You still need protection. What about AIDS?"

"What's that?" she asked.

She laughed in disbelief when I told her that sex could kill. Cloistered in the hospital for seven years, she'd never heard of AIDS.

The drive through Verdun was pleasant. Nancy filled me in on other Perry 2C gossip: her roommate had been transferred to another ward; Patrick was spending a lot of time in the side room. Et cetera. Nancy's chatter stopped when we veered onto the Bonaventure Expressway. I assumed she was taking in the scenery, the Montreal skyline she was seeing for the first time in a while.

"Slow down!" she shouted.

I jumped at the force in her voice.

"We're on an expressway, I have to keep up," I replied, a little miffed by her commanding attitude.

"How long have you been driving?"

The guileful tone of her question ticked me off. I pulled into the passing lane and pressed hard on the gas. Nancy banged her fist on the glove compartment.

"You're driving recklessly!"

"How would you know?" I asked. "You don't even have a driver's licence."

I sped faster to drown out the nasty rebuttals from the passenger seat. It never occurred to me that Nancy was unaccustomed to expressways, speeding cars and overnight passes. I slowed down only because I remembered the baby in my belly.

Twelve long minutes later, we turned off Sherbrooke onto rue St.-Denis. I steered into an empty spot between two cars. Nancy unbuckled and opened the passenger door before I'd finished parking. She stepped out and mumbled something about being tortured. I grabbed her overnight bag and joined her on the sidewalk, flustered from the drive.

"Welcome to our humble home!" Phil bellowed from the doorway.

"She almost killed us," Nancy said.

Phil and I exchanged glances. A long night lay ahead.

We sat down for dinner at seven, two hours later than Nancy's hospital schedule—an error on my part to veer from her routine. Nancy was hungry and cranky. Hospital dining had impacted her eating etiquette. Rather than lifting the fork, she bent forward over the plate and shovelled pasta in her mouth. I made nagging remarks like "sit up" and "slow down" and "put less pasta on your fork." She ignored me as I had ignored her in the car. After dinner, Nancy pushed Phil and me away from the sink and insisted on cleaning up, a long ordeal that took a great effort on her part, out of practice I assumed. She placed the last dish on the drying rack and collapsed on the temporary bed we'd made for her on the living room sofa. It was eight o'clock.

"Want to watch television?" I asked her, unsure what to do next.

"No."

She looked uncomfortable the way she had landed on the sofa, her legs twisted to the side. She stared without blinking at the ceiling light fixture.

"How about a magazine?" I asked.

"No."

I covered her with a wool blanket that used to belong to our parents, tiptoed across the room and flicked off the light switch. The "good day" had come to an end. Unaccustomed to being off the ward, she was likely exhausted.

"I'm not sleepy!" she called out.

She shot up from the sofa and marched down the hall. I turned the light back on.

"Nice of you lovebirds to sleep in a double bed and give me a crappy sofa," she yelled from the kitchen. Furious, I started after her, but Phil held me back.

"Let her be," he whispered.

Cupboard doors in the kitchen opened and slammed shut. Nancy was drying and putting away the dishes she'd washed. Phil went to the bathroom to pee. A huge crash and the sound of shattering glass. Nancy appeared in the doorway. Her eyes were wild and darting. She marched across the living room to where I was standing, a broken wine glass in her hand. We were miles from the side room, from nurses with syringes filled with sedatives. Sparks flew up and down my spinal cord, an urgent message to take flight. I refused to budge. My sister would never hurt me. The illness didn't scare me. She stopped abruptly, two feet from where I held space.

"Please give me the glass," I said calmly.

She stepped a little closer. Her lungs were wheezing with asthma.

"It was an accident," Nancy hissed and handed me the glass, the unbroken end.

She stormed back into the kitchen and called 9-1-1. Twelve minutes later, two medics showed up at our door. They asked Nancy what was wrong. She ranted in garbled franglais and insisted on being driven back to the hospital. The medics didn't understand. I tried to explain, but Nancy was yelling. The younger of the two looked a little bewildered. The older one touched Nancy's arm and asked if she needed help to walk. I handed over her spring jacket and overnight bag and he escorted her to the ambulance, her arm crooked in his. Phil lowered the blind to block our curious neighbours. I curled up in a ball at one end of the sofa and cried for a long time under the weight of our parents' wool blanket. When I woke, Phil was asleep beside me. The broken wine glass I'd left on the living room floor had been cleared away. The overnight pass had been a huge mistake, the evening a catastrophe. Nancy would spend the rest of the night in the side room. I should have driven slower on the expressway, not chastised her eating habits at the dinner table and let her sleep in our double bed.

For three days, my belly was unusually still. We rushed to the clinic for an abdominal exam. All is fine, they said. Even then, I was unable to relax. I roamed the apartment in a shitty mood for a week, snapping at Phil every few minutes, not realizing how bad I was feeling or why, a pattern that would repeat over the years to come.

The overnight catastrophe was safely in the past by the time my daughter entered the world in early August. A six-week-old baby was a beacon of light on Perry 2C. News travelled fast on the ward. Within minutes, the staff had congregated in the nursing station to have a peek at Nancy's new niece, Sarah.

"This is the baby?" Nancy asked from the doorway.

Hospital rules forbid patients to enter the nursing station uninvited. I walked over to Nancy and unwrapped the receiving blanket so she could see the wiggling little fingers. Sarah grabbed her aunt's thumb and made gurgling noises.

"Can I hold her?" Nancy asked, her dewy eyes on the baby.

I shrugged. Two nurses and an attendant had just held Sarah. Why not her aunt?

Nancy cradled Sarah in her arms and planted a long kiss on her forehead. A circle of patients formed around us. Nancy rocked the baby, radiating love.

"My baby," she said, beaming at the others.

Mr. Malik spoke up from the nursing station.

"I believe you mean *my niece*."

119

"My baby," Nancy repeated.

"Nance, please pass Sarah back."

I had spoken softly. Inside I was screaming. I reached out my hand that was shaking a little and gently squeezed Sarah's tiny foot through the soft cotton. Nancy stepped back, no intention of letting the baby go. My throat constricted, sandpaper dry, and my eyes started to sting. Phil would never forgive me.

Mr. Malik clapped his hands three times. "Shoo-shoo everyone, this is not a show!" He flapped his arms and the crowd dispersed.

"Nancy, give your niece back to your sister." His voice rang sharp with authority.

Nancy glared at me. Her eyes were on fire. She unwrapped herself from the baby and stormed down the hall towards her room, muttering obscenities. Sighs of relief came from the nursing station.

Mr. Malik unlocked the door. The baby viewing was over.

"Wait for me!"

Richard was scrambling down the hall towards us.

"Slow down," Mr. Malik called out to him. "What's the rush?"

"September 25, my birthday. Nancy's sister promised a kiss."

I clutched Sarah against my chest and leaned forward to kiss Richard's cheek—a quick peck on sticky skin—then stepped into the second-floor corridor. The steel door slammed shut behind me. Sarah babbled with excitement, oblivious to her mother's tears. I hoped that Nancy would be spared the side room. Maybe a small sedative would be enough. Not her fault to fantasize about a different life than the one delivered by genetic fate, the fate I'd been spared. I was a slippery fish, the sister who'd got away.

I woke on New Year's Day with a resolution and a throbbing headache even though I'd drank only two glasses. Over the years, my tolerance for red wine had become unpredictable, as had my patience with Nancy. The smallest exposure to either could trigger an unpleasant reaction. I liked red wine. I loved my sister. Both could make me miserable. To some people, the obvious solution would be to remove the red wine and the sister from my life, a vow I've often made at the height of anguish— and later retracted when I felt better. Some might describe my behaviour as self-inflicted abuse. Those people haven't a clue.

Keith brought me two Tylenol, a tall glass of water and my phone.

Nancy was disappointed when I cancelled our coffee date at her Benny condo. Everything was closed New Year's Day; she had nothing else planned. Sarah offered to step in even though she had made plans to visit some Montreal friends before heading back to Toronto the next morning. She, like her brother, grew up with her aunt's mental health struggle. My children's compassion and empathy for Nancy are deeply rooted.

The Tylenol knocked me out. I slept for two hours and woke up rested, the wine migraine gone. I was making tea when Sarah called.

"How did it go with Nancy?" I asked.

"To be honest, not great."

"Why? What happened?"

"I told her about the traffic and that the roads were icy, but she still complained about me being late. And she got mad when I had to leave. She said the visit was too short."

I sighed. Sarah hadn't seen her aunt in a while. I'd hoped their visit would go better. It sounded like business as usual.

"Yup, that sounds typical."

"Also . . ."

"What sweetheart?"

"She complained about you, Mom. A lot."

My back straightened. "What did she say?"

"You don't want to know."

"You're so right. Don't tell me."

"I won't." Sarah's voice sounded choppy, like she was close to tears.

"What's wrong, honey?"

"She was so mean about you, Mom. And you do so much for her. It's very upsetting."

An angry red sea swept over me. Sarah was still talking. I didn't follow her words. My vision blurred and my breath quickened. My temple started to pound. How dare she upset my daughter, who had so little free time and had gone out of her way to visit. This was unacceptable. I needed to protect my children from this goddamn motherfucking illness.

16

SPRING 1997, FORTY-TWO-YEAR-OLD NANCY was still stuck in a sedated holding pattern at the Douglas Hospital: thirteen years and counting. Meanwhile, Phil and I had moved back to Westmount. Our cozy townhouse below Sherbrooke was a world apart from where we'd once lived up the hill with our respective parents, a step down, my father might have said. I was determined to raise our young family in a calmer environment than frenetic rue St-Denis. I had enough chaos in my life with hospital visits, administrative affairs for my parents and a growing marketing business. Clients appreciated my strategic focus on realistic goals, an approach I had failed to adopt for myself. Friends called me "Super Susan," made of steel. Only Phil noticed how my forty-year-old armour was starting to rust.

A hospital social worker called during weekday morning mania. Sarah and Willy were bouncing in their chairs, waiting for breakfast. I turned from the noise, cupped my hand tight over one ear and pressed the phone against the other.

"Can you repeat that?" I asked.

"Your sister is being discharged."

I reached for my mug and took a gulp to steady myself. The coffee was cold and thick, hard to swallow.

"Are you still there?" asked the social worker.

My heart was fluttering. Nancy released?

"Yes, sorry. I'm a bit stunned. She's been at the Douglas for a long time—"

"She's responded well to the change in medication. The doctors feel she is ready to leave the hospital."

A few months earlier, Nancy had started Clozaril, a last-resort medication used when other antipsychotics have failed. The medication could trigger a life-threatening immunity condition called agranulocytosis. My sister's white blood cell count was monitored every four weeks. The drug worked like magic, lifting the fog from Nancy's brain. Her thoughts were no longer jumbled and her mood lightened. She was less agitated, able to engage in conversation. My parents and I were heartened by the unexpected progress, but our enthusiasm was dampened by the past. How long would these good days last?

"When is this happening?" I asked.

"I'm working on the discharge plan this morning. Your sister is first on my list."

"Do our parents know?"

"I wanted to check with you first. I understand you and your sister are close."

I blinked. Where in my sister's file did it say we were close?

"Nancy and I were raised in a quiet family."

The social worker laughed. "Your sister isn't exactly quiet now."

"I mean it was just the two of us. Not sure that means we're close."

Sarah tugged the back of my shirt. "We need breakfast, Mom. Look at the time. We're gonna be late." She tapped her fingers on the table.

Willy joined in, a monster-sized grin on his face.

"We want toast! We want toast!" they cried in unison, ignoring my waving hand, a weak attempt at discipline.

"Is there a possibility she could move in with you?" asked the social worker.

The question took me by surprise.

"Move in?"

"Do you need time to mull it over, discuss with your family perhaps?"

A sofa bed in my home office accommodated my sister's occasional overnight passes. So far, we had circumvented a repeat of the broken wine glass incident. The tiptoeing and emotional restraint was draining and disruptive to our family routine but a small sacrifice given the lousy deal my sister had been dealt. Moving in, on the other hand, was a different story. I pictured Nancy with the kids at the kitchen table. She wouldn't be tapping her fingers on the table. She'd be slamming her fists.

"I don't need time to mull this over," I replied. "The answer is no."

Four mornings later, on April 10, 1997, the social worker steered my sister out of the ward, down the stairs and into an office off the main hall of the Perry Pavilion for what my sister describes as a televised exit. She was about to re-enter society. Her "coming out" coincided with the latest round of Quebec government cutbacks and further deinstitutionalization of provincial health care; the Douglas Hospital was under pressure to reduce the number of beds. My head was muddled with questions, ones that still float in my brain. Did the budget slash influence the doctor's decision to prescribe my sister a last-resort treatment? Could she have taken the drug earlier, thereby triggering an earlier discharge?

The social worker delivered Nancy to a home in LaSalle owned by a couple with two young daughters. The residential neighbourhood was unfamiliar territory, farther south and west than the Douglas, ten miles from me and everything else. Nancy called in a panic, wondering what to do with her time. Except for art therapy on Tuesday mornings, she'd been discharged without a program, disastrous for someone who'd been bolstered by a strict regimen for thirteen years. The social worker apologized. Budget cuts had curtailed outpatient services. Nancy was lucky to have two hours of art therapy. "The host family will keep an eye on your sister," the social worker promised. This was part of the agreement they'd signed.

Sunday afternoon, Nancy was waiting for me on the front steps of her new home.

"How's it going?" I asked.

She looked up and down the street.

"I have no idea where I am," replied my sister.

We descended a carpeted staircase to a finished basement that accommodated three lodgers. Nancy's room was orderly and clean, single bed, dresser and chair. Lace curtains had been pulled across a ground-level window.

"It's a view of nothing," she said, watching me.

We sat side by side on the bed, facing a Monet print of water lilies. The room smelled like lavender potpourri.

"Now what?" I asked.

Nancy took me on a tour of the basement—laundry room, bathroom and two closed doors belonging to her new roommates. They were rarely home, she said. I followed her back up the staircase to a small living room filled with Ikea furniture. Raymond and Maria scrambled up from the sofa. Their handshakes were soft and warm. They had just returned from church. Raymond's tie was unknotted, the top button of his denim shirt undone. His black pants looked freshly pressed. Maria wore a green corduroy dress with black tights. Their two daughters, in matching frilly pink dresses, sat on the living room carpet, their long dark curls spilling over paper and crayons. Maria explained that her mother, who lived with them on the main floor, was lying down. Nancy had told me that the old woman was incoherent and spent most of the day on a custom-made potty in the bathroom off the kitchen. Maria had a full plate. Perhaps this explained the half-moons under her eyes. Hopefully, what the government was paying her to take in three former psychiatric patients was worth the effort.

Maria showed Nancy the bus route to the LaSalle Metro station and brought her to Costco for the weekly grocery shopping. Nancy joined in family outings to the park, to the cinema, to the ice cream parlour. Maria prepared the meals but gave Nancy free access to the kitchen. Perry 2C had roughened my sister's ways. She unhinged a cupboard door, broke two plates and burnt the bottom of a stainless-steel pot. Maria called me, stressed out. Her tone brightened when I promised our father would pay for the damages. The bill angered our father; "What did they expect?" he asked. Nancy called me daily, bored and restless. Better than the hospital, I reminded her. She was in good hands. My visits dwindled to every two weeks, sometimes three.

Nancy had been living in her new home for five months when I dropped by during a September heat wave, a last gasp of summer. The carpeted staircase smelled musky and damp. A dehumidifier was roaring in the basement hall. Nancy closed the door behind me. She pulled off the quilt and yanked at the sheets. The mattress was stained with urine.

"We had waterproof protectors on Perry 2C," she said. Her head bowed in shame.

My gut clenched. At forty-three, my sister was experiencing incontinence.

"It's not your fault that the pills knock you out," I said softly. "Dad can pay for a new mattress."

"Will you ask him for me? He might get upset."

"Sure, I'll ask."

"I have something to tell you," Nancy whispered.

"I'm listening."

"Raymond likes me."

I rolled my eyes. "Duh, of course he does."

"That's not what I mean."

"What then?"

She looked down at her lap. "We held hands."

I pictured Nancy with the family on the way to Dairy Queen. She steps off the curb without looking. Raymond grabs her hand and pulls her back.

"What's wrong with holding hands?" I asked.

Nancy frowned. "You don't understand. It was romantic."

A psychiatrist had once labelled her flirtation as "sexual transference." He said it was normal for a patient to fantasize about therapists and caretakers. I had a different theory. Her truncated adolescence and extended stay in the hospital had deprived her; she was man-hungry, a serious flirt, even with my husband. Harmless and understandable. Normal!

"Oh, come on. Don't go there. He's married."

Raymond's deep laugh penetrated the bedroom from the kitchen above us. He was on a week's holiday from work, Nancy explained, and bored out of his mind. I yawned, fatigued by our pointless conversation.

"What's the big deal? He held your hand."

"He kissed me on the sofa."

"Excuse me?"

"Maria and the kids were out shopping. I was feeling out of it, alone. I started to cry. He joined me on the sofa and took my hand. I felt better, like magic. Then he kissed me."

I didn't believe her. She was delusional and desperate for a boyfriend.

"Did you enjoy it?" I asked, studying her face.

"I felt uncomfortable."

Not the answer I had expected. My sister's story became more credible.

I followed Nancy into the kitchen. Maria was bent over the stove. Raymond was alone at the table; his daughters had vacated the kitchen and were watching cartoons in the living room. He looked up and smiled. A black leather jacket hung on the back of his chair; a pair of Ray-Bans was tucked in the breast pocket. Nancy sat down across from him and picked up a fork. She was eyeing me closely. I shifted my feet uneasily, my sister's steadfast advocate.

"Would you like to stay for lunch?" Maria asked. She had the slouch of an older woman.

I made up an excuse. Nancy accompanied me to the front door, the fork still in her hand.

"What should I do?" she asked.

I kissed her on the cheek. "I'll take care of it."

Back home, I left an urgent message for the social worker. Two hours later, she appeared on my doorstep with my sister and a suitcase. Maria called that evening. Her voice was high-pitched and full of venom.

"Everything we've done for your sister; how dare she accuse my husband."

"I'm sorry this happened." My voice quavered, teetering between reason and emotion.

"Your sister's a horrible person. She's trying to ruin our lives."

My back arched. Nancy was not the enemy. She was a victim. Surely, the monthly government cheque compensated for a few bumps. What if Raymond wasn't innocent? Nancy was attractive and vivacious, not worn down by house and family like his outraged wife. I steadied myself.

"You're putting me in a very awkward position," I said coolly.

Silence.

"I'm her sister. I have to take her side," I added.

She hung up on me, a final blow. My heart burned from the crossfire. Any sympathy for Maria vanished in a puff of smoke. I wasn't concerned about my sister either. She was back in civilization, a thirty-minute stroll from downtown. The only person I felt sorry for was myself.

The social worker was confident that a group home spot would soon become available in the Notre-Dame-de-Grâce neighbourhood as per our request. Six weeks passed. "Would you consider LaSalle or Verdun?" she asked at the end of October. I declined despite the massive disruption to our household. Nancy's previous experience in LaSalle had taught me the importance of a central location. She needed to feel connected. Meanwhile, my work had fallen behind, the kids ran wild, the house was a mess and Phil had resumed smoking. Another week passed. My parents invited Nancy to the Laurentians for a few days before their return to London in November. I jumped at the opportunity to drive her to their cottage, anything to expedite the event.

Our parents' driveway was covered by fallen leaves. Nancy, next to me in the passenger seat, had fallen silent.

"What's up, sis?" I asked.

"I won't be able to sleep and eat when I want."

I laughed. "That's for sure. Makes my home look easygoing, doesn't it?"

I reached over and squeezed her hand. The isolation of the cottage still gave me the creeps despite the beauty of the lake. I felt a twinge of self-doubt leaving Nancy behind.

Our parents had been overly optimistic about the visit. Inevitably, she clashed with their strict doctrine that had remained steadfast over the years. Our mother and father took turns calling me, unloading their complaints. Nancy had no table manners. Nancy slept too much. It was as if no time had passed except the voices sounded older, worn out.

Sarah and Willy were at the park with the babysitter when Nancy returned. She opened the rear passenger door, stepped onto the sidewalk with her bag, stumbled up the stairs and passed through the front door without saying goodbye to our parents, whose faces were strained and clouded with disappointment. My father joined me on the sidewalk. Mom remained buckled in the front seat.

"Do you want to come in for a cup of tea?"

My parents rarely came for a visit. They preferred to meet at a restaurant or wait for me to drive up to the cottage. Was it because of Phil that my parents avoided my home? Or were they not thrilled about being grandparents? My mom always asked about the kids in her letters from London; face to face, she was less enthusiastic. She had once confessed to never wanting a family. Why would grandchildren be different?

My father declined my offer for tea. He was anxious to return to the cottage before dark, an understandable excuse. I considered applying a little pressure. Sarah and Willy were due back from the park; they would be thrilled to see Granny and Pom-Pom. My parents' car pulled away from the curb. I cheered myself up with the thought of the cozy family that Phil and I had created.

Nancy was stretched out on the pull-out sofa bed in my office, snoring at foghorn volume. An hour later, I was still on the same page of a marketing report when the kids exploded into the house, followed by the babysitter's ineffective whine. The kids clambered up the stairs and burst into the office. Their live-in auntie still held novelty status in their excitable minds.

"Don't wake her!" I whispered.

Nancy rolled over and pulled the blanket over her head. Sarah opened the overnight bag and dumped the contents over her shrouded aunt.

"Oooooh. Pink candy!" Sarah cried and tossed a pill bottle in the air.

Willy picked up a wallet.

"Moneyyyyy!"

I pushed up from my desk.

"Kids, stop messing with your aunt's things."

Nancy growled from under the blanket, which stirred the kids even more.

"A monster!" they cried.

They bounced around Nancy and the contents of her overturned bag. I looked on, horrified by the cruelty of my children. They'd spent their first few years visiting their aunt at the Douglas. Had nothing seeped in?

"YOU'RE BOTH GROUNDED!"

The kids started to whimper. The babysitter appeared in the doorway. The vacant look in her eyes annoyed me.

"Take them away," I said and closed the door.

Willy was on the other side, whimpering.

"I'm sorry, Mommy."

I opened the door, hugged him, and closed it again. Despite the noise and hoopla, Nancy had fallen back asleep. The cottage visit had exhausted her as well as our parents. I returned the pills, wallet and other items to her bag and picked up the phone. My message recorded on the social worker's voicemail was brief and to the point.

"If you don't find a home for Nancy soon, you'll have two sisters to place."

Miraculously, a spot opened up in a Notre-Dame-de-Grâce group home managed by a woman named Mona.

"We know it's crowded with seven residents, not ideal. We'll keep looking," the social worker told me.

Nancy was indifferent. The kids were disappointed. Phil and I were overjoyed. After almost two months, our lives would return to normal.

Trouble surfaced a week into the new living arrangements. Nancy described Mona as the "Iron Lady." She ruled over the group home like a sergeant major, not surprising given the number of residents and limited space. Nancy invited me over, even though visitors were discouraged. The apartment was on the ground floor of a triplex. Mona, who lived in a room at the rear, was out buying groceries. Nancy showed me the padlock on the door to her room that she shared with two others. They were only allowed in their rooms after dinner. The kitchen was small and clean. Another padlock hung on the fridge door.

"We're not supposed to hang out in here," she said.

"Where's the bathroom?"

"This way."

The door was closed. Nancy knocked lightly.

"Go away." The man's voice was gruff.

"Someone's always in there," Nancy said, pinching her nose.

She pointed at the morning shower schedule taped to the door.

"If you miss your time, you miss your shower."

"You could always shower at our place."

She narrowed her eyes.

"That's not very practical. Want to see the living room? It reeks of cigarette smoke."

I shook my head. I'd seen enough.

A new round of discussions with the social worker filled the space in my life that had opened following Nancy's departure. Persistence paid off. Nancy was moved to a second-floor group home a block west from Mona's, one without locks and with only three residents. The owners lived on the ground level, delivered meals three times a day, cleaned weekly and were otherwise absent. I rested easy, knowing Nancy's freedom was restored. A minor glitch—one of the residents, a pretty thirty-five-year-old named Cathy, had threatened revenge on Nancy when they were both patients on Perry 2C. They'd had a run-in, Nancy told me: about what, she didn't say. Cathy looked harmless to me.

In late November, while the couple who managed the group home were out for dinner, a neighbour reported loud shrieking coming from the second floor. When I arrived on the scene, Nancy was sitting on the outside front steps wrapped in a grey blanket. She showed me the nasty swelling on her right leg and pointed up at Cathy's blank face looking down from the second-floor window.

"Your sister's tough," the paramedic told me. "She doesn't want to press charges."

I sat down on the step beside her. She was staring at the ambulance. Her eyes pulsated from the flashing light.

"Maybe you should get your leg looked at," I said gently.

"I'm not going in that ambulance."

The paramedic was right. My sister was tough. She'd endured intramuscular injections, electric shock, body restraints and the side room. She wasn't fussy about food, where she slept, sharing a bathroom or showering without a curtain. She could withstand a hard kick in the shin. The threat of being sent back to the hospital, however, was unbearable. She shivered under the paramedic's grey blanket and I snuggled closer, hit by a sudden wave of fatigue. Three group homes in less than one year, and my sister still hadn't found a stable one except for mine. We crouched together on the cold cement steps, ignorant of the turn of events about to take place. The next phase of our sister-lives would be relatively smooth and stable, a longer run than either of us could imagine.

Twenty-four hours after Sarah's unpleasant New Year's Day visit with her aunt, I was still fuming. Determined to take steps to protect my children from any further emotional dumping, I arrived at Nancy's condo complex and pressed down hard on the buzzer in the lobby. She let me in without asking who it was, which worked into my plan to catch her unprepared. I flew up the stairs and yanked open the fire door on the second floor. Nancy was hovering outside her unit at the far end of the hall. On seeing me, she called out.

"Yoo-hoo, Sue!"

Her friendly welcome slowed my feet. She was in a much better mood than I.

"You should ask who it is before you buzz them in," I said coolly.

"Darling, I knew it was you!"

How could she have known it was me? My visits to her condo were infrequent. We usually met in cafés, on a street corner or at my house. Still, I believed her. My sister didn't have friends who would just pop in like I had. A little pang tapped against my chest. She looked so happy, reminding me how my parents rarely stepped inside my home. She pulled me inside.

"My dentist appointment was cancelled. I didn't know what to do today. You've saved my life! Take off your boots. Let me take your coat. I'll make us some of the tea you gave me. You know, the turmeric one."

A second little pang.

She hung my coat in the hall cupboard and bustled into the kitchen. I lingered by the front door, unsure of my next move. I certainly hadn't come for tea. The wooden floors were gleaming and the air smelled like lemon furniture polish. Nancy filled the kettle with cold water. Her kitchen sink and the counters were spotless. The illness had not affected her clean and orderly ways. I crossed the floor towards our parents' rattan sofa and chair that had not been moved since I'd dragged them in here with Willy four years earlier. Her artwork still hung in the same places on the walls, including the painting by our mother that Nancy complained about. She had added her own touches to the room, notably the eye-catching throws and afghans she had woven at L'Atelier that were draped over tables and the backs of chairs.

I lowered onto the rattan sofa. The foam underneath felt even harder since my last visit. I'd recently read that dust mites and their detritus can double the weight of a mattress in a decade. The one I was sitting on was fifty years old. Nancy often mentioned that the sofa made her wheeze. I was always too busy to replace it. With shaking hands, she placed the teapot on the two-person mid-century kitchen table, a gift from me. She would have preferred less faddish, more solid furniture. I bolstered myself with the knowledge that my sister lived independently thanks to me. Otherwise, where would she be? The thought made me shudder. Nancy carefully poured the tea into two mugs. If it wasn't winter, I would suggest we sit on her balcony with the sweet view of the garden across the street. As I leaned towards her to pick up a mug, my rage dissolved. My daughter needed protection, but my sister needed it more.

17

DECEMBER 1998. A YEAR HAD PASSED SINCE the string of group home disasters that had ambushed my sister. We sat across from each other at a long banquet table in the Kensington Presbyterian Church hall. Our table, like nine others, was covered in a red vinyl cloth that would later be wiped down for future use. The place settings were adorned with forest green paper napkins, candy canes, chocolate angels and wooden dreidels. The evening marked Nancy's second Christmas-Hanukkah celebration with L'Abri en Ville, a charitable organization offering alternative housing for people with chronic mental illness. Promoting independence, connection and community integration struck me as a mainstream housing solution, not an alternative one.

Nancy no longer lived in someone else's home, nor did she share a room. She was one of three residents in a spacious, second-floor duplex in Notre-Dame-de-Grâce, one of ten homes managed by L'Abri en Ville. I'd learned about the apartments from a former Westmount neighbour, Julie, who hired Nancy to babysit before and after the first breakdown. Julie was not intimidated by mental illness; she had full confidence in my sister's ability. One of Julie's sons passed away at twenty-two, complications related to schizophrenia. Tragic. He'd been living in a group home at the time. Julie, a community-minded person, was aware of the importance of living in a safe and supported environment. Surprisingly, the social worker at the Douglas Hospital had never heard of L'Abri en Ville.

Nancy popped a piece of candy cane in her mouth and turned to the apartment volunteer on her right, a senior administrator with the provincial education ministry who accompanied Nancy to a community pool once a week. Beside him, the executive director of a local food bank shared a joke with Nancy's roommate, Geoff. I counted close to seventy volunteers in the church hall. They formed teams for each apartment, acting as mentors and friends to the residents, who often were disenfranchised from family. I was one of the few blood relations in the room. Geoff passed me the dinner rolls. Like me, he had a bachelor's degree in commerce from McGill. He'd once worked as a financial planner. His buttoned-down shirt and tie looked like a second skin.

"When do you think we'll eat?" I asked.

"Are you hungry?"

"Not particularly."

He smiled. "Good thing."

I should have known from last year's holiday dinner that we weren't eating anytime soon. Nancy's other roommate, Carlos, winked from the opposite end of our table. It wasn't a coincidence that my sister lived with two men. L'Abri en Ville staff had learned early on about Nancy's insecurity with women, especially younger, pretty ones, and, more to the point, her yearning for a romantic relationship. Carlos had a soft heart and twinkling eyes. A short-order cook, he'd been saved from the street by L'Abri. He was friendly but kept his distance, a smart move on his part. Romantic relationships were strictly forbidden among roommates.

I locked eyes with the president of the board at our neighbouring table. An elegant woman in her late sixties, she had dressed for the occasion: a red knit suit, lipstick and dangly silver earrings. Straightening my grey wool blazer that hid the black T-shirt I'd been wearing all day, I noticed a dark stain on the lapel, one my fingernail could not scrape off.

"Try soda water," Geoff whispered.

Geoff was one of the original members of the family at L'Abri and the mainstay of the apartment. Every Christmas, he served a turkey dinner for a small gathering of L'Abri en Ville residents who had nowhere to go. This year, Nancy was thinking of joining them instead of coming to our house.

"Did you buy your turkey?" I asked.

Geoff put a finger to his lips and pointed to the stage where the president was now standing, a dinner bell in her hand to silence the festive chatter bouncing off the church hall walls. She called the residents and volunteers to the food table, one apartment at a time. Finally, our turn

arrived. Nancy filled her plate with sliced turkey, stuffing, scalloped potatoes, roasted carrots and green peas. She passed on the gravy as our
parents always did. I scooped up a few potatoes and peas. The church
hall did not inspire my appetite.

"Vegetarian?" asked a tall man with longish greying hair standing behind me in line.

"Sometimes," I replied. My response sounded silly, even if it was true.

"If you're not into turkey, I strongly recommend the spinach lasagna.
It's delicious."

His articulate manner of speech and scruffy-formal appearance suggested academia, but I knew better than to presume. His name tag gave
no clue if he was a volunteer or resident, a welcome change from the
top-down hierarchy of a hospital or group home. Under his supervision,
I helped myself to a modest portion with the intention of sharing with
my sister. The aroma of fresh garlic, tomato and Parmesan stirred my
appetite. I returned to the table and ate everything on my plate. All that
was missing was the glass of red wine waiting for me at home.

"Can we leave after this?" I whispered to Nancy.

"There's more to come," she said.

Staff announcements followed, then the residents were invited to
speak. Nancy's hand shot up in the air. She stood up, proudly wrapped
in a stunning shawl she had recently finished, her first woven art from
L'Atelier. In a clear and unwavering voice, she recited a poem about her
experience with L'Abri en Ville, with humorous rhymes that triggered
giggles in the audience. She concluded on a serious note: "I thank my little sister for all she does for me." Nancy beamed at the applause; I fidgeted
with discomfort. L'Abri en Ville was the one to be thanked. And Julie.

A middle-aged woman in an ankle-length black dress and clunky
snow boots climbed onto the stage and thumped across the wooden
platform towards a cello secured on a stand. She lowered unsteadily onto
a small stool and folded forward over the instrument. Long wisps of
dark hair curtained her face. I'd heard a rumour that she used to perform
with the Montreal Symphony Orchestra before her illness. She swept a
bow across the strings: J.S. Bach's *Brandenburg Concerto*. I closed my
eyes, transported to the twinkling lights of a cavernous cathedral during
our family's 1960s holiday in London. I had complained profusely to our
parents about going inside another old church, the same feeling I had
about attending a second L'Abri en Ville holiday party. The four of us had

settled in the back row of the cathedral just as a string quartet began to play. Our father had leaned over and whispered, "J.S. Bach's *Brandenburg Concerto No. 3*."

Nancy's shoulder brushed against mine, bringing me back to the present. She reached for my hand, which she held until the end of the cello performance. I wanted to ask her if she remembered the string quartet in the cathedral, but I never had a chance. Our table had been called up to the dessert table.

Relieved by their daughter's stable living situation with L'Abri en Ville, our parents invited Nancy to stay with them in London for two weeks. "Are you sure?" I asked. They were insistent and Nancy was thrilled. A vacation! She hadn't been overseas since my plunge into the River Thames. On the day of her departure, I arrived at the apartment well in advance of the flight. The apartment door was wide open. Geoff stood in the entranceway with his arms crossed. A suitcase was on the stairwell landing.

"I bet that bag's been packed for days," I said, grinning.

He nodded.

"Has she been driving you crazy, Geoff?"

"I've been spending a lot of time in my room with the door shut."

"Smart idea."

Geoff unfolded his arms and stepped closer.

"I lodged a complaint at our weekly meeting, just wanted you to know."

"Complaint?"

"Your sister insists on taking out the garbage and recycling at four in the morning, even if it wakes us up."

"Does she know about the complaint? She hasn't mentioned anything."

"She was sitting next to me on the couch at the time."

"How did she take it?"

"She said some nasty words and stormed out of the room."

Geoff's hands were shaking a little.

"I'm sorry."

"She doesn't respect our house rules."

"Let's hope the trip does her some good," I said, trying to be positive.

He leaned closer. "I'm curious; was she always like this?"

I didn't feel like hashing through the past. I patted his shoulder.

"Her trip will be a break for you and Carlos."

Geoff refolded his arms and tapped his elbows. "Her medication needs to be changed."

Nancy had told me about the stacks of pharmacology books on his bedroom shelf. Geoff was well-read on the subject.

"Do you think drugs can fix bad behaviour?"

His eyebrows arched.

"Of course."

A door slammed inside the apartment. Nancy appeared behind Geoff.

"You didn't tell me my sister was here. Geoff, I need help with my bag!"

Her soprano voice spiralled down the stairwell. I flattened myself against the wall on the landing to give Geoff room to pass with the suitcase. Nancy and I followed him to the street and watched as he heaved the bag into my trunk. He waited on the sidewalk while Nancy and I buckled up. I lowered the window and waved as we pulled away from the curb.

"Bon voyage!" Geoff called.

I looked over at the passenger seat. My sister was shuffling items in her bag, unaware that Geoff was waving.

"Say goodbye to your roommate, Nancy!"

She lowered her window and waved.

"He's a good guy," I said. "Helping you like that."

"We're good to each other."

I waited until we were on the expressway to share what was on my mind.

"I understand you take out the recycling very early in the morning."

She banged her fist on the glove box. My timing sucked. She was nervous about travelling, easily triggered.

"They're all against me!"

"Calm down. No one's against you."

"Don't you tell me to calm down!" she shouted.

"Lower your voice, please. It's dangerous when I'm driving."

She fisted the glove box a second time.

"I'll shout if I want!"

My grip on the wheel tightened. I had organized the airline ticket, purchased and delivered the suitcase, checked in with Dr. Byrne and put up with her frantic calls the last two weeks. I didn't expect a reward, but I didn't deserve to be yelled at. I turned on the radio and cranked the volume. Nancy opened the passenger window and blasted me with cold, angry air. I fumbled with the window controls. The car swerved a few feet into the passing lane.

"Close your goddamn fucking window!" I shouted.

"Turn off your radio!"

She won. I turned it off.

"Now close the fucking window!"

She paused, her finger on the switch.

"Now!"

Finally, she relented.

A message flashed on the dashboard. The front passenger door was open. I glanced sideways. Nancy's hand was on the door handle.

"Jesus Christ, your door is open!"

"I was going to jump out," she said sullenly.

"That's ridiculous. You would never do that."

"How do you know?"

"I know."

"Why are you slowing down?"

"Because I can't drive with the door like this. What if it flies open?"

"It won't."

"How do you know it won't?"

"How do you know it will?"

No place to pull over, I put on the flashers and eased off the gas. Cars raced by in the passing lane.

"When I give the okay, open the door a little and then close it."

We slowed down: 70, 65, 60, 55, 50.

"NOW!"

She banged the door shut. We sat in silence, recuperating.

I veered onto the airport departure ramp and drove up and down the rows of parked cars, ignoring Nancy's complaints about arriving late. We finally found a spot at the far end. The wheels of my sister's suitcase clicked across the asphalt and through the revolving door. The terminal was buzzing with action. Nancy made a beeline for the British Airways counter like a seasoned traveller. I trailed behind, wondering why I hadn't just dropped her off. She handed the ticket agent a white envelope with Dr. Byrne's letter authorizing her to bring medication on the flight and declaring her mentally fit for travel. The agent read the letter while playing with a strand of streaked pink hair. She handed the envelope back to Nancy and turned to me. Her eyelashes were thick with mascara.

"Is she okay to fly alone?"

Nancy had been instructed to show the letter only if asked.

"My sister is fine. Our parents are waiting at the other end."

The ticket agent smiled.

"How sweet to escort your sister."

"I don't need a sister escort!" Nancy cried.

"Let's get something to eat," I suggested, hoping to calm her turbulent mood before takeoff.

We sat at a table littered with crumpled napkins and used packets of ketchup and mayonnaise. Nancy unzipped her carry-on and rummaged through papers—passport, boarding pass, Dr. Byrne's letter.

"Relax. You've checked everything three times already."

She spread her English money over the table.

"Should I go to the gate soon?" she asked.

In 1999, there were few amenities once you passed airport security. "What's the hurry? You can't board for another three hours."

"I'd feel better if I was at the gate."

"Order something. It's a long overnight flight. What do you want?"

She pushed the menu aside. "Grilled cheese. You sure it's okay to bring my meds on the plane?"

"If anyone asks, show them the letter."

"The letter! Where did I put it?"

I flagged down a server and ordered. Nancy continued to organize.

"This isn't a grilled cheese," she said when the food was delivered.

"It wasn't on the menu. I ordered you a club with cheese. Pick out the meat if you don't want it."

"What kind of restaurant doesn't make grilled cheese?"

I bit into my sandwich, starving. Nancy stood up. "I'd like to go."

"Can you wait for me to finish?" I asked, my mouth full.

"This isn't about you. This is about me."

She picked up her carry-on and hurried out of the restaurant towards the security line. I threw a $20 bill on the table and ran to catch up.

"Were you going to leave without saying goodbye?" I asked, out of breath.

"Of course not."

I wrapped my arms around her and squeezed. Her fingers fluttered over my back, barely grazing my skin. I squeezed harder, for the both of us, and then retreated to the other side of the roped fence. The line inched forward. Nancy was chatting with everyone. She disappeared behind the frosted glass wall without a final wave.

The London visit would be a resounding success, to be repeated every March for several years. Our parents were grateful for their daughter's company. Nancy was grateful for the excitement of a London vacation. I was grateful for the weight L'Abri en Ville had lifted from my shoulders. I dismissed the altercation in the car and the complaint Geoff had lodged. Those were L'Abri matters, not mine.

I brushed the snow from the windshield and started the engine. Nancy, in short sleeves and leggings, was supervising from her second-floor balcony in the -5° weather. I signalled for her to go back inside. She stepped closer to the railing and waved. Pleased with our relaxed visit, the taste of turmeric tea still on my lips, I drove down Benny and turned onto Sherbrooke with a smile on my face. Sarah's unpleasant conversation with her aunt had been filed away along with all the other unpleasant encounters.

Before going home, I drove to the Metro Westmount parking lot to stock our near-empty fridge with healthy food, another New Year's resolution. I pushed through the turnstile and headed for the fresh fruit. An elderly woman in a knit hat and wool coat approached me in front of the bananas. She told me that we'd met ten years earlier when my sister and I had addressed the Unitarian Church Sunday congregation. I remembered the event very well. Nancy and I had stood elbow to elbow at the podium, holding our prepared script that described her long struggle with mental illness and her search for a stable home that had led to L'Abri en Ville. At the end of our presentation, we bowed to a teary audience and then fled to the reception hall in search of food. Congregation members intercepted us, shook our hands and shared their own stories. The woman chatting with me in the grocery store had told us a heart-wrenching account of her thirty-year-old son, who had stopped taking medication and refused to leave her house. She didn't have the heart to kick him out. He had nowhere to go.

I lowered five bananas into the cart and asked about her son. The woman bowed her head. She trembled as she explained that he had drowned in the St. Lawrence River. Accident or suicide, she didn't say. I stood with her until she steadied, the least I could do. Her suffering made my complaints trivial. She gave me her number, which I stuffed in my coat pocket.

Back home, I unpacked the groceries and made a strong coffee to boost me for a writing session. Instead, the caffeine made me jittery and restless. I worried about Sarah working too hard in Toronto, Willy's latest job filming from a boat in the middle of the Pacific Ocean, Keith alone at the cottage. An email from Nancy's landlord flashed on my screen. Nancy's building manager had recently sent a warning about leaving garbage in the hall. I clicked on the message in a panic. The last thing I needed was to find Nancy another home.

But the email was about me, not her. Nancy's January rent was three days late; I had forgotten to transfer the funds. Was there anything wrong, the landlord asked. I read the email three times, an admonishment for my negligence. How could I forget to pay, a simple click of a button? I remembered the woman in the grocery store, how her face was drawn tight by guilt. She had complained of her son when she'd first spoken to us at the church. And now he was gone. My kitchen window rattled from the wind. Another winter storm was coming. My sister sometimes forgot to lock her balcony door. A gush of air could blast it open, not life-threatening, but the cold air could trigger her asthma, which was life-threatening. I stepped away from my desk to call her.

18

FORTY-FIVE MINUTES NORTH OF MONTREAL, the temperature dipped below zero and the fields bordering the Laurentian Autoroute were coated in a sheet of icy snow. The mountains in the distance sparkled with hoarfrost. I passed the exit for la Porte du Nord, where Sarah and Willy used to order french fries and burgers to spare them from the sardine and smelly cheese lunch at their grandparents' cottage. At eleven and nine years of age, the kids no longer accompanied me. Three days earlier, my parents had returned from their London sojourn. My sister had flown back with them, concluding her second annual visit. The morning after their arrival, the Laurentian region was hit by a massive snowstorm, not a complete surprise in a province known for winter in spring. My father advised postponing my visit, but I'd already rearranged my tight schedule to free up an afternoon.

A few miles north of Ste-Agathe-des-Monts, the autoroute merged with a divided highway. The pavement looked suspiciously dry. I tapped the brakes lightly as a test. My rear wheels jammed over the black ice and the car fishtailed towards the ditch. Feet off the pedals and steering like mad, I returned the car to the middle of the lane. For the next fifteen minutes, I drove slowly with the four-way flashers blinking, the muscles in my back and neck working overtime. Finally, I arrived at the exit, a tricky left turn across the highway. I waited for a break in the oncoming traffic, all the while praying that the traffic approaching from behind wouldn't smash into the rear of my car. Once the left turn was completed, I pulled over to catch my breath before continuing the last stretch of the journey, a dirt road with hairpin turns, deep ditches and no cellular service.

My hands were still trembling when the front door of my parents' cottage swung open. My father's seventy-nine-year-old face was etched with worry lines, some of them new.

"Thank God you're here. How were the roads?"

"Not bad."

We kissed on one cheek, English style, and I passed him a shopping bag stuffed with five months' worth of my parents' sorted mail.

"Where's Mom?" I asked, peering over my father's shoulder. She was usually with him to greet me.

"Lorna's getting dressed."

"At noon?"

"Our new routine."

He took my coat and carried my boots dripping with melting snow to the rubber mat. My mother scurried out of the bedroom and hugged me, a fleeting embrace, and then stepped back to inspect. I was wearing a wool sweater from Simon's, a deep shade of blue she would approve of. She tightened the sash belt on her housecoat, as if suddenly aware of her state of undress and disappeared back into the bedroom without an explanation. I thought nothing of it. Jet lag, probably.

A platter of food covered in plastic wrap had been left on the kitchen counter. My stomach growled with anticipation. Over the years, I'd grown accustomed to my parents' lunches. The familiar routine was comforting. My life had changed dramatically; my parents' lives had not changed at all, to my knowledge. My father lifted the wrap off the platter. The vegetables had been sliced and arranged, red alternating with green with my mother's artistic flair. Presentation is key, she once told me.

"Mom makes the best platters," I told my father.

"I made lunch," he said quietly. "Wine?"

"Sure."

He poured a generous glass, which he handed to me, and then raised his own.

"Welcome home, Dad."

We clinked glasses and sipped. My father pointed at the kitchen window.

"Lake's still frozen," he said grimacing. "Bloody cold."

"Same every year, no?"

"Yes."

"It must be hard to leave London when the magnolias are in bloom."

He winced. "It's always a shock to come back."

"Was it okay with Nancy?"

He brightened.

"It was a pleasure to have her. She was a tremendous help."

"Well, that's good news. How did she help?"

"Groceries. Vacuuming. Dusting. Lorna and I are slowing down. Well, maybe not so much Lorna as me."

"You look tired, Dad."

"I'm not sleeping well."

"Have you ever slept well?

He smiled. "Perhaps not. How are the children?"

I was surprised by the question. My mother was the one who usually asked.

"They keep me busy. Remember what I was like at their age?"

He shrugged. Maybe he didn't.

"Lorna loves the photos you send in your letters. She tapes them on the fridge."

"What photos?" my mother asked, walking into the kitchen.

"The photos of the children, darling."

"Children?"

"Sarah and Willy," he added.

"You don't need to remind me of their names."

"Sorry, darling."

"I'm not an idiot, Norman."

"No, you're not."

"Then stop agreeing with me like I'm an imbecile."

My father glanced at me.

"Shall we eat?" he asked.

I followed my parents to the dining room, dismissing the small argument that had likely started before my arrival. Before she sat down, my mother carved off a generous hunk of Camembert, which she popped in her mouth.

"Darling, leave room for some vegetables," said my father.

"I'll eat what I like," she snapped and lowered into her chair.

Five minutes later, my mother tapped her fork against the wine glass.

"Norman, you're taking all the cheese!"

"You already ate some, Mom," I said in his defence.

"Little Miss Smarty Pants."

Her words stung. I looked over at my father. His worried face was impossible to read. The scene reminded me of a tense meal with Nancy, her snarky behaviour when triggered.

"That's not a nice thing to say," I said coldly.

"I can speak to you any bloody way I like."

My mother's hard-boiled glare stopped my tongue. My father placed a piece of his cheese on his wife's plate, a peace offering. I bit into a cucumber slice and chewed longer than necessary, trying to make sense of the scene. My mother was always happy to see me after her long absence. We should be celebrating her return.

After lunch, my father took me aside in the kitchen.

"Your mother's having memory problems. We saw a specialist in London. He says it's a form of dementia."

My throat tightened. "Alzheimer's?"

"The tests were inconclusive."

"That's why you look so tired."

He shrugged. "The sleeping pills aren't working anymore. I'm up to a double dose."

I reached for his hand. The skin felt warm and dry.

"Shit, Dad."

"Shhh. She's coming."

My father limped out of the kitchen. His arthritic hip had worsened over the winter. He greeted my mother in the hall and placed his hand lovingly on her shoulder. She stared into the kitchen in my direction with the same stony look I'd seen during lunch. My father was right to be patient with her anger. Underneath, she was lost, confused and possibly terrified. I turned to the sink and blasted hot water over the dirty dishes, fighting back tears. Just when my parents and I were getting along so well, their lives were unravelling.

My mother's memory continued to deteriorate into the summer. She was no longer motivated to paint as she had been doing for the past twenty years. She skimmed newspaper headlines instead of reading novels. She refused to swim in the lake, even on sweltering July and August afternoons. More alarming was her irrational rage directed at my father when he engaged in his activities, especially when he practiced music. On several occasions, I witnessed my mother rushing into the living

145

room and pushing her husband aside. Capitulating to avoid a scene, he would slide to the far end of the piano bench and give his wife space to play the old hits from the '40s, the notes and lyrics still clear in her head. Ironicaly, she played better than ever. Even her singing voice, once rough from smoking, had improved. The mind and body work in strange ways.

My father continued to roll with his wife's moods even though they were wearing him thin. He ignored my suggestion to rent an apartment in the city, closer to services, closer to his daughters. He refused to budge from his long-standing routine, even if that routine was crumbling around him. Nancy joined our parents every weekend. Sometimes I gave her a lift. More often she rode the provincial bus. Eager to gain favour as she had in London, she mowed the lawn, helped with meals and watched over my father during his four o'clock swim. She didn't mind our mother's attacks; her skin was much thicker than mine. Our father depended on his eldest daughter's visits. I worried that she was spending too much time with them. Apart from her roommates and lunch dates with Julie, Nancy hadn't made new friends since her discharge from the Douglas, not even at L'Atelier where she wove Tuesdays and Thursdays. She did not respond well in most group activities, including those organized by L'Abri; too much competition for individual attention. I asked her about unstructured time during the week. Was it too much? She told me not to worry. The weekends at the cottage filled a social void in her life. I wasn't sure it was healthy. But then again, what did healthy mean for my sister?

Five months later, on a fading summer afternoon, I followed my father down the steep path to the lake. His hip was bone on bone, according to the orthopedic surgeon. He needed surgery. The pain was tolerable, my father said. His wincing suggested otherwise; he was afraid to leave my mother alone. Our descent to the lake was unbearably slow, more so since my mother had scrambled down the path ahead of us. The loss of short-term memory had infused her with a restless energy.

"Norman, do you have my bathing suit?" she asked when my father stepped onto the dock, puffing and flushed. His grimace transformed into a tender smile.

"Darling, you don't like to swim anymore."

She eyed the lake, choppy with whitecaps.

"Oh yes, I forgot."

I sat cross-legged, my towel folded underneath. The cedar decking was worn and full of splinters. My father had replaced some boards a few years earlier. Even those were looking old. Before leaving for London in November, he would drag the winch down to the lake to pull out the dock for the winter, a huge production that took longer every year. Thankfully, Nancy would help. My father adjusted his goggles, raised his arms, and bent forward. He never bothered to dip a toe to acclimate to the cold water. SMACK. He landed on the lake like a plank of wood and swam towards Dr. Navi's dock, four hundred feet from ours. The strength of his upper body propelled him forward; his feet kicked without purpose, barely breaking the surface. Like me, my father had never mastered the crawl.

"Aren't you going in?" asked my mother.

A chilly breeze prickled my bare skin.

"I think not."

"You should."

"I'll go in if you go in."

"Where's my bathing suit?" she asked.

"Do you want me to go up to the house and get it, Mom?"

"Naaaw, too cold."

My father circled back from the Navi's dock. He was losing steam, dragging his body towards us, determined to finish his four o'clock swim: a bloody-minded Englishman. He pulled himself up the ladder and staggered upright. The veins on the back of his legs were bulging. My mother applauded his return and asked for a refill. I filled the pewter glass halfway, the way my father had instructed. She tapped her foot and whistled, "All the Nice Girls Love a Sailor." The wine had lifted her momentarily.

I helped my father carry two sets of oars that he kept between two birches near the shoreline. We slid the fibreglass rowboats into the lake and tied both sterns to the end of the dock. My mother climbed into her boat with ease, my father less so into his. They paddled off in a westerly direction, my mother in the lead. I'd watched the performance a hundred times. On the return journey, they would switch positions, my father's boat in front, my mother's behind, their oars at rest. He would toss her a rope that she attached to a hook in her bow. If the wind was in their favour, and it often was, my father would open a golf umbrella, which he raised to catch the westerly breeze. They would sail back to the dock, two boats as one. Perfect symbiosis.

November came around again. London time. I drove my parents to the airport and ushered them to a table in the same restaurant where we always sat, as I did with Nancy on her annual departure in March. I had become part of their travel routine. My father repeatedly checked his documents, just like Nancy had done. My mother ordered a second glass of wine.

"Lorna, you've had enough, don't you think?"

She glared at my father.

"Norman darling, you can't possibly know what I think."

The incident forgotten, they hobbled over to security with their walking sticks, Norman leaning on his to support his hip. Like Nancy, he never looked back. His focus was on what lay ahead. Lorna, living in the moment, turned and waved every few steps, a silly grin on her face. Suddenly, she was lost, hidden by a group of young men in baseball caps. A blue hand appeared over the crowd, my mother's driving glove stretched over the handle of the walking stick she had raised three feet in the air. I guffawed, attracting the attention of a passing airport employee. My finger pointed at the waving blue glove.

"That's my mom," I said, tears of laughter rolling down my cheeks.

My parents disappeared behind the frosted glass. I turned around and walked blindly towards the terminal exit. For so long, I had wanted my crazy family to disappear. Now I wanted them to stay forever.

A year later, in the fall of 2003, my father was admitted to the Montreal Jewish General for a hip replacement. He had hoped to resume his life at the cottage after the standard three days in the hospital, but the surgeon insisted on a week-long rest at the Catherine Booth rehabilitation centre. Nancy suggested our mother stay in the Plaza Towers, a furnished apartment hotel on the eastern edge of Westmount. Our father was fearful about leaving his wife alone. "We'll take good care of her," I promised. How difficult could one week be?

I pulled up to the Plaza Towers. My mother was nowhere to be seen. I found her in the lobby, chatting up the security guard. They were laughing.

"What's the joke?" I asked.

"I forgot which apartment I'm in!" She was smiling, in a good mood.

My mother waved her walking stick at the guard and followed me down the ramp to the sidewalk. I opened the front passenger door and she peered into the back seat at Sarah, who was reading *Harry Potter and the Chamber of Secrets*. My mother jammed the seat belt into place.

"Are we going to see Norman?"

I turned onto Atwater. "He's being transferred to the Catherine Booth this morning. I thought we would drive to Beaver Lake instead."

"When can I see him?"

"This afternoon, maybe."

She pointed at the back seat. "What's *she* doing here?"

"She is your granddaughter, Mom."

"I know who she is. The question is, why is she here?"

"It's a pedagogical day."

"A peda what?"

"Ped-a-gog-ical. A day off."

"Doesn't she have any friends?"

"I have friends," Sarah said.

"Why don't you play with them instead of following your mother around?"

"That wasn't very nice," I muttered.

"*That wasn't very nice,*" my mother replied, imitating my voice.

I turned left on Sherbrooke, instead of continuing up Atwater towards Beaver Lake. My mother wouldn't notice.

"I'm dying for a coffee," she said when I parked in front of the house.

She was in a good mood again.

Sarah disappeared upstairs, out of harm's way. I steered my mother to the back porch.

"Have a seat. I'll bring you a coffee. It's a beautiful fall day."

I kept a close eye through the kitchen window, especially when our temperamental grey tabby, Buddy Love, jumped onto the porch railing two feet from where my mother stood. She started to play with the cat's tail.

"Fucker!" she yelled. "It bit me."

She raised her hand to knock the cat off the railing. I ran onto the deck and stood between my raging mother and the indignant tabby.

"Move aside. That damn Bloody Love thing bit me," she growled.

I shooed the cat off the railing and my mother stormed into the kitchen.

"Where are you going, Mom?"

"Somewhere I'm treated with respect!"

I followed her out the front door and onto the sidewalk.

"Mom, come back!"

She kept walking. I followed her up Claremont, keeping a safe distance.

She crossed Sherbrooke and turned left. I followed her three more blocks before she slowed down.

"Mom, this is crazy. Please come home."

"I want to go home. Where are my car keys?"

"At my house."

"And the car?"

"There too."

Thankfully, she had forgotten about the car by the time we retraced our steps. My parents' Subaru was safely parked in the garage under the Plaza Towers and my mother's keys were tucked away in my purse. I didn't mention the incident to my father when I took my mother to visit later that afternoon. Nor did I tell him it had been impossible for me to get any work done since his surgery. My mother required constant attention, far more demanding than Nancy had been in her most agitated state.

Our father performed his physiotherapy dutifully and was discharged from the rehab centre three days early, a miracle recovery for his age according to the orthopedic surgeon. They returned to the Laurentians, and I resumed my family-work routine exhausted and drained, ignoring Sarah's remarks about the crack in the living room ceiling. She was worried that her parents' bedroom, directly above, was about to collapse. I told her a twelve-year-old should not be concerned with adult problems. Her father and I would find a solution. She ignored my platitudes and pointed at the ceiling. "When will you fix it?" she repeatedly asked. The solution came six months later when, at my initiative, Phil and I separated. Nancy was not surprised. Mom and Dad never approved, she said. They knew this was coming. I didn't care what she or my parents thought. Walking away from a marriage was the one thing I could control.

I grabbed a handful of dirty socks from the laundry hamper and stuffed them into the one-inch gap along the bottom of the closed bedroom door. The barricade failed to muffle the swearing from the kitchen underneath. On hands and knees, I crawled along the carpet to the far corner of the bedroom and pulled my phone out of my back pocket. My fingers fumbled over the keys, entering the password three times before the music started, Bob Marley's "Exodus." I cranked the volume and hugged my knees. Keith's powerful voice still resonated through the floorboards.

Our fight had anesthetized my brain; I could no longer remember what had sparked the argument, what I'd said (or shouted) to trigger the quick temper Keith usually kept in check. The hall cupboard slammed and I lowered the music to listen; a wooden hanger fell to the floor, a zipper slid up his coat, boots thumped on the mat, the front door swung open and banged shut, the latch turned. Silence. I shivered with the memory of his face distorted with rage. A bough from the cedar knocked against the bedroom window reminding me of the unforgiving January night. I turned off the reggae music.

A marriage counsellor once told me it was healthy to argue. Nothing wrong with a little fighting, he'd said. He didn't understand that I'd grown up in a volatile household, that I'd withstood the bitterness of an angry sister who'd been dealt a lousy hand, that I'd reached the limit of my endurance. The slightest raised voice triggered echoes of discord in all four chambers of my heart. I suffered from anger intolerance, and yet anger was impossible to avoid. I hugged my knees tighter and studied the dark shadow under the bed, the perfect peaceful hiding place for a small child, not a sixty-year-old woman.

19

FORTIFIED BY MY DAD'S NEW HIP, our parents departed for London in time to watch the fifth of November Guy Fawkes fireworks from Battersea Park. Our father was neither religious nor celebratory, but he took pleasure in the annual toast to the failed conspiracy by provincial Catholics to assassinate the Protestant king. Our mother was happy to toast anything. Fortified by English bloody-mindedness, her husband steered them between continents for another four years until the winter of 2008, when their High Street physician refused to prescribe any more sleeping pills. My father experienced brutal spasms and extreme sweating from his sudden flurazepam withdrawal. At eighty-six, he could barely take care of himself, let alone his wife. He called me often from the flat, whispering that he was losing his mind. When I drove my sister to the airport at the end of March, I half-jokingly told her to bring our parents back alive. Nancy's presence was always appreciated in London, less so in her apartment where her unruliness was on the rise, as was my diplomatic intervention. I proposed that L'Abri write a letter of concern to Dr. Byrne; surely a medication adjustment was the solution. They kindly sent me a copy, which I read and then immediately filed, leaving the problems for the professionals to solve. (L'Abri was in charge, not me.)

Life at home was ramping up. My adolescent son sprayed graffiti and my eighteen-year-old daughter was rarely in sight—an even greater worry. Add to the list a second marriage to Keith, two teenage stepchildren, a massive home renovation and a marketing client who refused to pay a large invoice. To survive this time of mass confusion, I developed a virtual ticket system: a number one ticket was awarded to whoever needed it most, most recently my father, who'd been admitted to the Montreal General Hospital for evaluation less than a week after his recent return from London. My mother and I were stuck with each other, again.

The sky was still dark when I pushed up from the pull-out sofa bed in my home office. Keith rolled over, taking the blanket with him. The toilet flushed, followed by footsteps in the hall. My shoulders tensed, waiting for my mother to call from the other side of the door. I waited ten minutes, then tiptoed into the hall and peered into the bedroom. My mother's left hand dangled over the edge of our pillow-top mattress, revealing a wedding band loosened from age. The geriatric specialist had suggested she stay in a retirement home while my father was assessed at the hospital, perhaps at Place Kensington, a ten-minute walk from me. The appointment had not gone well. My mother had sworn at the manager and stormed out, nearly running into a bent-over lady pushing a walker. I stayed behind to apologize, then hurried to the lobby. My mother was nowhere in sight. I drove in circles until Geoff called to let me know she'd turned up at their L'Abri apartment—in a jolly mood, he said, with no idea who'd given her a lift but desperate for a cup of tea.

I closed the bedroom door and returned to my office, shutting that door as well. Keith was sitting up, rubbing sleep from his eyes. We'd discussed my plan for half the night. A glimmer of daylight flickered through the venetian blind. It was time for action.

Six hours later, the bathroom was a cloud of steam. I scrubbed the hospital dirt off my limbs until the skin turned pink and reached for the white fluffy towel, feeling such luxury was undeserved after what I had done. The front door slammed and my sister's voice rang up the staircase. Last night, she had kindly offered to distract our mother so I could work that afternoon. I hadn't yet told Nancy that the plan had changed. She was already in the upstairs hall when I opened the bathroom door, the fluffy white towel wrapped around me.

"Where's Mom?" she asked, looking into my bedroom.

"At the hospital."

"You left her alone?"

I braced myself against the bathroom doorway. "I have bad news."

"Oh no, is Dad okay?"

"He's fine. It's Mom."

"What's wrong with Mom?"

"She's been admitted."

"What?" Nancy's eyes opened wide.

"The doctor on 13East convinced her to go to emergency for a blood test."

"I don't get it. Blood test?"

"It was an excuse to get her into a hospital gown. They took her clothes away."

"How do you know all this?"

"I was in the room with her."

"Did she freak out when she realized what was going on?"

"They called a code white. It took four attendants to hold her down."

"Did they give her a needle?"

I nodded. "A big one."

"Did she ask for us?"

I shook my head. "She screamed for Dad."

My sister's eyes clouded over. With both parents incapacitated, she was suddenly rudderless, an orphan. I studied her face, searching for emotion: anger, sadness, resentment or grief. I found nothing. She took a step back and lifted her arm, as if saying "enough."

My eyes welled up with tears. "Please forgive me. I couldn't handle Mom any longer."

Nancy raised her arm even higher. Her blank face transformed into a huge grin.

"Revenge!" she shouted as our palms slapped together. We danced in the upstairs hall, bumping into walls and each other, eventually landing on the floor buckled over with laughter, a sister moment I will cherish forever.

Our diminished parents never said goodbye to their Laurentian cottage or the London flat. Their new life centred on a one-bedroom apartment in Place Kensington. I assured the manager that Norman would keep Lorna under control. Nancy and I agreed to split the visits, mine during the week and hers on weekends. For six months, we operated as a sister tag team, until the manager beckoned me into her office and asked me to sit.

She looked up from her desk with sharp, penetrating dark eyes that had served in the Israeli military.

"What's up?" I asked.

"We have a problem."

"Oh dear. My mom?"

The manager shook her head.

"Your sister won't be allowed to visit if she continues to be disruptive."

I knew what she was thinking. It runs in the family.

"What happened?"

"She ran down the hall screaming about your parents. Very disturbing for our residents."

"I'll have a chat with her."

"If it happens again . . ."

"I'll make sure it doesn't."

The manager eyed me. Her dark eyes softened and the corners of her mouth lifted into a small smile. "You carry a lot of weight for such narrow shoulders," she said. "You must be tough."

I thought about correcting her. I wasn't tough; I was trapped. I shrugged off the comment, more concerned about losing my tag team. My sister didn't fit into a conventional retirement home like Place Kensington—not now, not ever.

The meeting in the manager's office was a minor blip compared to the tumour in our father's colon, undetected during the battery of tests during his hospital assessment stay. The mass was successfully removed, but fluid from the bowel leaked through the stitched incision and triggered a life-threatening infection that called for an emergency colostomy. I paced the perimeter of a small waiting room while our father, dangerously weakened by two surgeries, lay intubated in the intensive care unit. Contrary to the surgeon's prognosis, Norman recovered (bloody-mindedness again). He returned to Place Kensington where, in his absence, Nancy had earned accolades from the staff for her endurance with our mother. With the parents back on track, I scheduled colonoscopies for Nancy and myself. Several polyps were removed from my colon, including one with high-grade dysplasia. My sister's procedure was aborted due to intestinal looping from chronic and drug-related constipation. She was given an appointment for a CT scan.

At this interlude, Keith insisted we leave for Costa Rica, a holiday we'd postponed for a while. Susie's turn for the number one ticket, he said. Two weeks at an eco-resort in the laid-back beach town, Sámara, flew by. On the last day, we inquired about Casa Verano, a white stucco, Spanish-style house directly across from where we were staying. The listing was overpriced, at least for our budget. Still, it was fun to dream.

Forty-eight hours following our return from Costa Rica, my sister and I waited in a microscopic examination room. Nancy's file with the CT scan results sat on the stainless-steel table.

"Do you think I have bowel cancer like Dad? Is that why they called me in?" she asked. Her face looked yellow under the fluorescent lighting.

I patted her shoulder. "I'm sure it's nothing."

My breath was shallow and my stomach a little queasy, like I'd felt when they told me about my pre-cancerous polyp. I wished the surgeon would hurry up. The room was stuffy, with no distractions except for a graphic poster of the gastrointestinal system tacked to the wall. Finally, the door opened. In marched the surgeon wearing a white lab coat. He opened Nancy's file and clicked on the keyboard.

"The colon is clear," he said.

"Yay!" I cried.

"Phew," sighed Nancy.

He pointed at something else on the screen.

"See that shadow on the pancreas?"

"Not really," I replied.

"Which one?" asked Nancy.

"It looks like an endocrine tumour."

Nancy started to weep. I uncrossed my legs and straightened.

"Is it malignant?" I asked.

"Probably," he said. "But it's the best kind of tumour to get: slow-growing."

The surgeon's eyes were fixed on me, even though we were discussing my sister's body. Despite Hollywood blockbusters and social media, mental health was still stigmatized, even within the health profession. I pointed at my sister.

"Not my tumour," I told him.

A smile cracked the surgeon's face. I hadn't meant to be funny. He turned to address Nancy.

"We need to get it out," he said.

Afterwards, in the hospital coffee shop, I reminded Nancy what the surgeon had said. "The best kind of tumour to get." Neither of us felt reassured. She played with her fingers, which looked pale next to mine. My heart ached for her, and for me. Another avalanche had hit, one that swept away the two weeks of Costa Rican *pura vida*. Had the trip been worth it?

The operation was scheduled quickly. I stayed with my sister until they wheeled her into surgery. She was in an upbeat mood, bolstered by the attention of two male attendants, one of whom led me to the family room where half a dozen people waited in a time warp. I tapped a pen against my journal and studied the perfectly shaped leaves of the tropical plant in the corner of the room. The man beside me sneezed without covering his face, my cue to move to the empty seat beside the tropical plant. I stroked a leaf. Plastic. Too fidgety to write, I returned the journal and pen to my bag and pulled out a *New Yorker* magazine. The egg sandwich the woman beside me was eating turned my stomach. I moved a second time and checked my phone. Thirty minutes had passed since my sister had been wheeled into surgery; four and a half hours to go.

The resident came for me mid-afternoon. The operation had gone well, he said. As a precaution, they'd removed two-thirds of the pancreas and all the spleen. I called my parents. They sighed with relief and asked when I was coming to visit. Not for a few days, I told them. Nancy held the number one ticket.

Nancy was the last patient remaining in the recovery room. The anesthesia plus the residue of the antipsychotic medication had made her unusually drowsy. She wouldn't be moved until morning,

"Can you stay the night?" asked the nurse at the recovery desk, a middle-aged man with a reddish complexion and dark-rimmed glasses. He shuffled papers for no apparent reason. Too much caffeine, perhaps.

I stared with incomprehension.

"Excuse me?"

"Your sister may wake up disoriented or agitated. We never know how patients like her might react to the anesthesia. You know, waking up in a strange place and all."

"She's used to hospitals. I'm sure she'll be fine."

"I've read her mental health history. It would be better if you stay."

Better for whom, I wondered. My sister or him?

Three hours later I returned to the recovery desk with a small overnight bag. "I was hoping for a king bed," I said to the nurse, eyeing the narrow cot beside my sister. He adjusted the IV and fled back to his desk, my joke lost on him. The recovery room was dark except for the fluorescent light over my sister. She looked angelic, a flicker of her former self. I removed my coat and boots and lifted myself onto the cot, wiggling under the thin flannel sheet, happy for my wool socks. I stuffed my hat and scarf underneath the pancake-thin pillow. Even with my eyelids squeezed shut, the fluorescent beam over my sister's bed was blinding. I pulled my coat over my face. The light faded, but still I couldn't sleep. I tiptoed out of the recovery room into the hall in search of a bathroom. One of the cleaning staff waved his mop at me. In my grey sweatpants and white T-shirt, I'd been mistaken for a night-shift attendant.

The day nurse woke me at dawn, a gentle nudge on my arm. Sunlight streamed through the wall of windows. The sharp smell of disinfectant stirred my foggy head.

"Where's my sister?" I asked, surveying the empty space where her bed had been.

"She's been moved to the tenth floor."

I dropped back on the cot and pulled the flannel sheet up to my chin.

"That was the worst sleep ever," I groaned, remembering the hundred times I'd rolled over.

"Sorry, but you have to leave."

Did the nurse really believe I wanted to stay?

For the next three days, Nancy's eyelids remained half-open, even when I turned up the volume on the portable radio I'd brought for her, even when I danced like a crazy fool. She picked at her meals, uninterested in the candy I'd smuggled into the room. Our conversations were limited to basic requests. Please get some water. Please take me to the bathroom. I need my toothbrush. On the morning of the fourth day, I collapsed in the visitor's chair, perplexed.

The doctor wasn't concerned when I insisted my sister wasn't acting her normal self. He said, "She's had major surgery and needs to rest." After multiple requests, the head nurse finally showed me the hospital medication schedule, which I compared to the list of drugs from Nancy's pharmacy. My sister's bedtime and morning pills had been reversed. No wonder she was groggy during the day. Lesson learned: I knew my sister better than any health-care worker.

On the fifth day, Nancy's eyes opened fully. She was in great humour, thanks to the pain medication. Her laughter bounced down the hall as she entertained the nurses, doctors, attendants and cleaning staff. She flung up her hospital gown to reveal a foot-long incision across her belly that would leave a Frankenstein zigzag scar, not for the faint of heart. She gobbled down her meals and asked for seconds, for juice, for another pillow.

The post-op holiday was short-lived. With reduced pain medication, Nancy became irritable and agitated. She complained about the food and the nurses. She barked at me, and at Geoff when he came to visit. I suspected something more was going on than physical discomfort. Her pain threshold was normally high; all those years in hospital had toughened her up. Her eyes darted around the room looking at invisible threats. Her fingers played with the wound, a reminder of her mortality. It struck me watching her that my dear sister had braved a sick mind for so long; a sick body scared her to death.

"Don't touch your belly, Nance. It'll get infected."

Her eyes narrowed into dark slits.

"Sweetheart, I'm already infected," she hissed.

The adrenaline that had fuelled my body for the duration of the five-week hospital stay fizzled out the morning after her discharge. A breath-stealing pain in my shoulder woke me. I couldn't move my right arm.

"Adhesive capsulitis," the doctor at the orthopedic clinic said. "Frozen shoulder."

He approached the examination table with a long needle pointed at the ceiling.

"This will hurt a little . . ."

I squeezed my left hand and counted. The doctor discarded the needle and washed his hands in the sink.

"Frozen shoulders often occur under extreme stress," he said, his back to me. "You don't seem the type."

I continued to count in my head, waiting for the cortisone to take effect. My stress was buried deep, far from public view, and the tension had erupted through a weak spot, my right shoulder, proving the manager at Place Kensington wrong: I wasn't as tough as I looked.

My arm regained mobility during the walk home from the clinic. I lifted my hand over my head. A young man in a black Mercedes waved, mistaking my gesture. I laughed out loud, a hearty guffaw that cleared the fog from my brain and turned my thinking in a new direction. I couldn't wait to share my idea with Keith. I arrived at our front steps, ravenous and energized.

Keith was thrilled with the new direction I proposed. Three months later, we were rocking back and forth in handcrafted leather chairs under the breeze of a whirling ceiling fan. The stone patio was a sanctuary in the afternoon when the heat restricted activity to sipping tea and turning pages of a book. Shadows from the bougainvillea danced across the cement wall separating our garden from the steaming jungle. In a few minutes, I would jump off the edge of the plunge pool, knees squeezed against chest, chin tucked. My body would hit the water in a perfect sphere, creating a tsunami from a cannonball. I would rinse off in the outdoor shower, maybe lounge in the hammock strung between two palms in our front yard. For breakfast, we'd eaten papaya and pineapple; for lunch, avocado and farm eggs. Dinner was too far in the future to contemplate. A deep groan echoed from the jungle, the same roar that had piqued our curiosity when we'd stayed at the eco-resort across the street. Black shapes appeared near the top of a guanacaste tree, the howler monkeys' afternoon swing-by. I pinched myself for the hundredth time. My low bid for Casa Verano had been accepted. We were living the dream, if only for a few weeks at a time. Keith appeared with two mango juices and an invitation for a boat tour. Friends were easy to find ten degrees north of the equator.

An hour later, I crawled onto the bow and raised my chin at the sunset, a middle-aged figurehead on an old fishing boat. We turned from the mainland and met the incoming waves head-on. I gripped the gunnels and squealed at the salty spray. A sudden cool breeze turned my head. Behind us, the full moon peeked through the Cordillera de Guanacaste.

I pointed at the sinking sun.

"*Mas rapido*! Before she disappears!"

"Crazy Canuck!" our friend shouted. He knew what he was talking about. A former investment advisor from Toronto, he hadn't worn shoes in years.

The sun dropped below the curved horizon, into another world. Our captain steered towards the coastline. Once moored, we waded over stones and shells. Four of us climbed onto a two-person quad, no rules in this remote village. We navigated around the expats, avoiding the potholes. The Costa Rican road was rough but smoother than the one I'd left behind.

We rested a day before our next adventure, a waterfall unmarked on the tourist map. I followed a young Tico up a thirty-foot precipice, reminding me of a younger self who climbed trees. My heart was beating strong, like the bow of the fishing boat hitting the waves. The Tico youth reached the summit and dove headfirst into the river. I stepped into his place and looked down. My daredevil son's whisper, all the way from

Montreal, urged me on.

"Go for it, Mom!"

I smiled with my son's impish grin and jumped off, arms spread wide like wings, heart freed from responsibility.

Mid-January and I was sick of snow. Sick to bloody hell of it. The view of the mountains from our Eastern Townships cottage was pretty, beautiful even, but void of life. I missed autumn when the leaves prepared themselves for their release from the branches. The colours in the landscape were still vivid back then. I missed forever summer in Costa Rica even more. Keith joined me at the window and wrapped his arms around my waist, pulling me in.

"Perfect day for a snowshoe," he whispered in my ear.

I rubbed my finger. "Think I'll pass, thank you."

"What's wrong with your hand?"

"My finger's stiff, hard to bend."

Keith poked me gently. "Maybe you're getting old."

The joke annoyed me. The stiffness wasn't from age; it was from winter. I continued to stare at the mountain landscape even though the black-and-white expanse had nothing to offer.

"I need to go back to the city."

The city had distractions—stores, buildings, cars and people.

Keith frowned. "What are you going to do there? Apart from visit Nancy?"

"Dunno. Maybe see a friend."

"I don't believe you."

He was right. I had no energy for friends.

"Look," he said. "We're still new in this community. When spring comes, your life will pick up, like it did in Sámara."

"You just want me to stay so you have company."

The hardness in his eyes told me I'd spoken too harshly.

"Do what you want," he muttered, walking away.

I returned to the bleak landscape and crossed my arms. A friend had advised against selling Casa Verano despite our many reasons. Too hot, too many bugs, too far, too expensive, too much hassle. We had lived the dream and then the dream ended. "Costa Rica holds you and Keith together," our friend had said. He was right in a way. The heat placated us. We didn't argue for six winters. The cold northern reality was a different story. The cottage was a secondary home, not an escape. Sadly, I had learned in the tropics that all escapes are temporary.

Keith touched me lightly on the shoulder. How long had he been standing there?

"What can we eat for lunch?" he asked brightly. He was fighting his mood. Mine was too far gone to fix.

"You go ahead, I'll eat later."

He squeezed my upper arm with affection, like a parent would.

"I know you. You'll have coffee and a cookie for lunch."

I smiled and said nothing.

"I'm not sure what to eat . . ." Keith's voice trailed off.

"Take the rest of the chicken from last night. And the sweet potatoes."

"Good idea," he called on his way to the kitchen.

The tops of the mountains were cloaked in clouds. White flakes circled the house. Soon, the temperature would drop. The roads would be covered in ice. If I stayed any longer, I risked being stranded in a winter-bound marriage that needed attention I was unable to give. The last thing I wanted was another person to watch over, another responsibility. Being alone was the only way to take care of myself. I turned from the bay window and followed Keith to the kitchen. The sooner I left for the city, the better.

20

I NODDED AT THE EVENING NURSE to administer the morphine drip. My mother's eyelids fluttered and traces of foamy spittle leaked from her mouth. I leaned over the intravenous tubing and promised to take care of my father and Nancy, soothing words in a room that reeked of antiseptic and death. My promise would be easy to keep; it fit into what I was already doing. The bony grip on my hand relaxed. The nurse placed two fingers over the radial artery and checked the clock over the bed. My eighty-nine-year-old mother had passed two hours before winter equinox 2012, the end of the world according to people who believe in Mayan mythology. For them, she had left just in time.

I was worried about my sister's reaction to our mother's death. What would this unleash in her mind and in her behaviour? Would it trigger a psychotic episode? Her response was surprisingly calm. She cried for a minute, a quiet whimper. Then wiping her eyes, she asked practical questions. What had the hospital done with the body? Where would she be cremated? When was the funeral? I didn't have any answers, distracted by the onerous task of breaking the news to our father. Nancy and I both knew the job fell to me. We agreed I would tell him first thing in the morning. She would meet me at Place Kensington. I couldn't sleep that night, haunted by the anguish on his face that would slice my heart into pieces. My turn for grieving would come later.

On the day of the funeral, a severe winter storm blasted Montreal. Nancy called it our mother's last stand. With our father sandwiched between us, we trudged through eight inches of snow towards the dark blue awning of the funeral home. Two blank-faced attendants in three-quarter-length coats greeted us at the double wooden door. They'd been trained not to smile, not to frown.

Once inside, we removed our winter jackets. My father wore his navy suit and a silk necktie he'd owned forever. Nancy and I were in black. We were directed to a small chapel populated by a sprinkling of friends and L'Abri volunteers, more mourners than I'd expected given the storm and holiday season. I sat with our father in the first row, next to Keith, Sarah and Willy. Nancy chose a seat farther back, closer to her L'Abri family, not that she stayed sitting for long. Her excitable chatter from the aisle drowned out the farewell playlist I had arranged. She made a joke about being at a cocktail party. Our father stared straight ahead at the porcelain urn that housed his wife. He scowled and lifted his nose in the air like he smelled something unpleasant, the perfume from the white lilies perhaps. He asked if we were in a church. "I didn't think you wanted a church; this is a funeral home," I whispered. He remained silent. I comforted myself with the thought that my father would be miserable regardless of the arrangements. I stroked his hand, bony like my mother's. His fingers stayed perfectly still, no response to my touch. He didn't need a morphine push; he was ready to leave. I wish I had known that at the time.

Keith, acting as the funeral officiant, stepped up to the podium.

"Hey, Keith, is that stained-glass window behind you real?"

The audience cracked up at Nancy's rhetorical question. The window was as fake as the chapel. Keith responded to his sister-in-law's inquiry with a deadpan delivery and then invited me to speak. Nancy moved farther down the aisle, three rows closer to the podium. She was gearing up for more wise-cracking comments. My eulogy would not go undisturbed. I wanted to throttle her, inflict bodily harm, interrupt her poem when it was her turn. Of course, I failed to act on any of the above and admittedly, when I picture her straddling the aisle in that gloomy chapel and playing the crowd while I delivered my sombre speech, I can't help but smile.

Three months later, I orchestrated a different kind of funeral, one that began with Keith tapping a spoon against his glass. The guests looked up from their conversations and fanned into a semi-circle, facing a floor-to-ceiling window with a view of the pond that had served as a skating rink three weeks earlier. The restaurant at Mount Royal's Beaver Lake had been a destination of our father's during his Place Kensington years. Nancy and I stepped into the semi-circle. I was dressed in grey linen pants and a button-down white blouse. She wore a turquoise dress. We faced a crowd of fifty, their eyes at half-mast from the spring sun streaming in through the wall of glass. I recognized Mr. Malik from Perry 2C. He'd aged little in twelve years. Two first cousins, a brother and a sister on our father's side, were standing far apart, as they did in real life. Nancy recited a clever stream-of-consciousness rant she had composed and I sang "Little Brown Jug" by Joseph Eastburn Winner, an old tune my mother loved to play on the piano and my father loved to hear, especially the part about being pickled in alcohol, the closest my parents came to discussing death. Speeches concluded, we invited the guests to the buffet table, where platters of sushi were displayed between framed photographs of our father at various life stages: Royal Navy officer, meteorologist, business executive, retired traveller. Nancy popped a spring roll in her mouth. I hovered over the platters, unsure. Loss had affected our appetites in different ways. Keith handed me a glass of Riesling. I cringed at the sweetness, just like my father would have done.

"I want to go home," Nancy said, her mouth full of sushi.

"We can't leave yet. We're the hosts."

"I need someone to drive me."

"Give me a minute. I'll call a taxi."

"I don't want to be driven by a stranger."

"Can you wait half an hour? Maybe Keith can drive—"

She turned before I'd finished my sentence, marched to the far end of the buffet table and joined a small circle of L'Abri family. At that moment, I was of no use to her. The loss of our father so close to our mother had triggered the reaction I'd feared three months earlier. Without the anchor of a parent, even an ailing one, my sister had become unmoored. Tension in the apartment was running at an all-time high, especially on the weekends when Nancy no longer had a parent to visit and run errands for. I hoped the storm would blow over with a medication adjustment or two.

Meanwhile, my father had been gone only ten days, and I was already drowning in a sea of paper to sort out his estate. The funds Norman Grundy had left in trust for his eldest daughter had mushroomed into an administrative nightmare that would keep the lawyers and accountants occupied for three years, surely not my father's intention. I tried my best not to complain about my privileged problems. The testamentary trust, once settled, would take care of my sister for the rest of her life, sparing me financial burden. My life, however, would be less burdened if I had a healthy sibling to share the load. The long-ago wish I'd made to be an only child continued to bite me in the back. I should have wished for two sisters instead of none.

Julie, who kept close to Nancy since she had joined L'Abri, waved her car keys. I sighed with relief. Nancy had found a lift home, one less thing to worry about. I took a second sip of Riesling and turned to the window. The sky over Beaver Lake shone the same brilliant blue as it did over Casa Verano, only twenty degrees cooler. I wiggled my toes, remembering the sand.

The following January, Keith and I abandoned our parkas and snowboots for an extended three-month stay at Casa Verano. Keith was semiretired and I had reduced my workload to a couple of contacts that were manageable from a distance. Nancy was not pleased with the plan. What would she do without me all winter? I purchased an iPad and showed her how to FaceTime. We'll be able to see each other, I told her with enthusiasm. She banged on random keys, half-listening to my instructions, or more precisely, not listening at all. The day of departure, I purchased a long-distance plan for my cell phone. At least we would be able to talk.

Our first morning back in Costa Rica, I dropped in on a writer's group I'd read about on a community Facebook page that described Sámara as *the Black Hole of Happiness where the longer you stay, the less you'll want to leave.* The writers assembled at a vegan restaurant, Luv Burger, every Wednesday morning. A vivacious woman with tattooed arms and silver bangles approached me and introduced herself as Danya. She smelled like coconut and eucalyptus and her mane of dark curls was pulled high on the back of her head. She asked if I knew anyone. I waved at the sunburnt English expat named George, who liked to drink despite his heart condition. His red Liverpool FC jersey from last winter looked a little faded. Danya asked if I had brought a piece of writing to share. Butterflies fluttered in my chest. I scanned the seven middle-aged expats, all strangers except for George, and he knew very little about me. What did I care what these people thought about my writing, good or bad? I flipped through my journal and stopped at an untitled piece I'd been playing with, an amalgamation of my sister's words and mine.

My guarantee ran out when I was thirteen. A host of powerful emotions pulled me in all directions. Keeping up with other kids was exhausting. It was difficult, then impossible, to concentrate on homework, television, and conversations at the dinner table. Thoughts grew more bizarre. I was afraid to confide in anyone. How could I explain what I couldn't understand? I lay awake for two nights. The summer heat hung over my bed like a suffocating blanket I couldn't kick off. At dawn I cut off my hair with my mother's sewing scissors.

Benztropine made my tongue thick and slow. I drooled and my belly grew. They sent me home for a while. I misbehaved. My mother would get upset and cry. My teenage sister was running around with her friends. My father tried to reason with me. Kids were cruel, teachers not much better. I graduated from high school and then university after many hospitals stays.

I paused to take a sip of water. George had dozed off. The man beside him in Bermuda shorts and a wild-patterned shirt was making notes in a book, likely last-minute revisions to his writing. An older woman in a wide-brimmed straw hat and orange-patterned kaftan flagged down the server. Danya was the one person looking at me. I regretted not reading something else.

I lived my thirties and some of my forties in a locked ward at a psychiatric institution. Mention the name and people look uncomfortable. I was one of the lucky few with visitors. At first my sister came alone. Then she brought a baby. Then she brought another.

This reflection is depressing. Thank God, I'm due for an antidepressant in a couple of hours. Joking! Maybe my story sounds worse than it was. Hard to say: I don't know anything different. The good news is that I was released from the locked ward by a new drug and I live in a real apartment with kind people who watch over us. I'm turning sixty soon. I suspect that the tumour they removed from my pancreas was from the new medication.

The surgeon said I had a lucky break they found it. I call it good bad luck. Twice a week I weave. People say I have a good sense of colour. When I sit at the loom, it's like I'm playing the piano. I could have been a concert musician. Or a ballerina. Instead, I hang out at Dollarama and McDonald's. I talk to people—sometimes I know them, mostly I don't. My sister warns me not to talk to strangers. I do what I want.

My parents are gone and my sister still runs around like a teenager even though she has wrinkles—more than me. I admit feeling jealous. She gave me an iPad for Christmas thinking we could stay in touch. She spent hours telling me how to use it, a waste of time. That's my sister's world, not mine.

I closed my journal with an unintentional whack. George opened his eyes.

"Not finished," I said. "Just a draft."

Danya thanked me for sharing and shuffled papers. Her bracelets clunked against the table. George straightened his back. The silence made me uneasy. I played with my pen, then folded my arms. My writing wasn't great. Still, I'd hoped the piece would trigger discussion or, at the very least, a comment.

George cleared his throat.

"My mother was schizophrenic. It was hell."

"Something to write about, perhaps," I said quietly.

Danya asked the man in Bermuda shorts to read. I lost the thread of his story, distracted by George and his mother. In the weeks to come, George would share a great deal about his childhood.

The older woman in the straw hat and orange kaftan approached me on the beach later that afternoon. She said I was brave to tell my story and that I had managed a serious illness very well. I started to explain and then stopped. What did it matter? No judgement in this beach town. I left my sarong and flip-flops under a palm tree and ran towards the water. The soles of my pale feet smacked against the hard-packed sand. The ocean was calm, a disappointment to the novice surfers who flocked to Sámara for the waves. I swam out thirty feet, farther than usual, and rolled onto my back. My mother was easy to find in the cumulous clouds.

She was facing me, gliding on her belly, a big grin on her face. Her legs broke free and took the shape of a grand piano. My father's fingers curled over the keys. They glided out to sea, oblivious of their youngest daughter watching from below. My sister was nowhere to be seen in the clouds, still bound by the earth, not even an ocean between us. The thought weighted me. I kicked my legs and flapped my arms to stay afloat. A sharp stone grazed my lower back. I stood up awkwardly in knee-deep water, surprised that the incoming tide had pushed me so close to shore. I washed the cut with salt water and remembered my neighbour's infected foot. From bacteria in sea water, she'd said. The sarong stuck to my wet skin as I hurried up the road in search of Polysporin and a bandage.

The aching stiffness in my right middle finger became more pronounced, whether I was alone in Montreal or with Keith at our mountainside cottage in the Eastern Townships. Heat provided no relief, disproving my theory that winter was to blame. I struggled to tie bootlaces and zip up my coat. One morning, I could no longer open the mayonnaise jar that Keith had screwed so tight. "It's from all that writing," Nancy told me when I showed her my third finger that could no longer bend. I disagreed. The stiffness was as bad, sometimes worse, on non-writing days. A more likely culprit was *accumulated busyness.* My hands never stopping caring for this, caring for that. Keith called my finger a rigid digit. I called it an angry finger, stuck in "fuck you" mode. With a simple twist of the wrist, I could easily make a peace sign. But I didn't feel very peaceful. I resigned myself to the stiff and useless finger, one more aspect of my life that I could not control.

21

THE DIRECTOR OF L'ABRI EN VILLE FOLDED his hands over the vintage oak desk donated by a generous volunteer. His fingers were long and slender, and his nails looked professionally manicured, quite the opposite of mine. Beside him, on the windowsill, three pots of geraniums sat in a tidy row. The plants were bursting with foliage and flowers, a marked contrast to the bleak late December sky. I fiddled with a painful hangnail on my thumb, waiting for the director to tell me why I'd been summoned. His request for a meeting during the Christmas holiday was not an encouraging sign, nor was the thick manila folder placed front and centre on his desk. The cover was stained from a coffee spill. The corners were dog-eared.

"Sorry I missed the holiday dinner at L'Abri," I said, anxious to end the awkward silence.

He waved off my apology.

"No worries. You're allowed to take a break," he said.

I laughed to myself. A break? The passing of my parents almost three years earlier and the recent departure of Sarah and Willy from the nest should have freed up my schedule. Instead, I was bogged down with sister problems, even though Nancy was still under L'Abri en Ville's care.

The director reached for the manila folder.

"Your sister's file," he said.

I giggled, a nervous response.

"That's a lot of paper," I said. "Nancy's been with L'Abri forever."

The director crossed his arms on the desk and leaned forward.

"We've been dealing with problems for quite some time."

He flipped through the file. Nineteen years of my sister's life fluttered up from the pages.

"It's all been documented," he said.

I looked away from the file. The thick fleshy leaves on the geraniums reminded me of the climbing hibiscus in our little garden at Casa Verano. In a week, I would be shooing that damn iguana from eating all the flowers.

"There've been a few bumps since our parents died," I said quietly.

"More serious than bumps, I'm afraid. And the problems have been going on long before that."

I turned back to the director, his file. A sharp pain jabbed my temple. The fluorescent lighting in the office was suddenly harsh.

"The problems didn't seem that serious, at least not until recently," I said.

"We didn't want to burden you."

I massaged my forehead to ease the ache.

"Is the situation that bad?"

"Yes, that bad. You must have noticed as well?"

I played with the silver chain hanging from my neck. Last September, against everyone's advice, I'd fulfilled a promise to bring Nancy to London for two weeks. The trip was a disaster, even though I'd had the support of Keith and my first cousin. Fourteen days of verbal abuse and constant demands left me with a phantom lump in my throat and the sensation of being strangled. I couldn't wear anything around my neck for months. My doctor called the condition globus pharyngeus. You'll get over it eventually, he said, and then asked if I'd learned my lesson. My doctor knew Nancy well. He was her doctor, too.

The director continued.

"Nancy's been threatening Geoff. Yelling and shouting in the apartment. Yesterday, she clapped her hands in front of his face and spat. We do not tolerate aggression. She's already had two warnings . . ."

I was aware of the two warnings. Each one had sent Nancy and me running to Dr. Byrne for a medication adjustment to address her rising agitation. Last month, he'd written a note to buy her more time. It read something like this.

November 4, 2015: To whom it may concern: This is to attest that Nancy's recent increase in agitation and irritability has been related to side effects of recent medication changes. I am redressing this, and Nancy should return to her baseline functioning in a matter of weeks.

Eight weeks later, my sister still hadn't returned to her baseline. Had her medication stopped working or was the illness spiking? By now, I understood enough of the malady not to bother asking Dr. Byrne. He didn't know. Nobody did. He had prescribed a low dose of Latuda, an antipsychotic, with the hope that Nancy would respond as so many of his patients had. Unfortunately, she did not. Nancy's case continued to be a hard one to crack.

The director was staring again. He had his agenda; I had mine. My mind raced to pull together a winning strategy. I would rally support from L'Abri's board of directors. My sister was a long-term resident. Surely, that counted for something. Dr. Byrne would back us up. Maybe if he increased the Latuda . . .

"We need more time," I said.

He shook his head.

"I'm sorry. This is a final decision. Nancy must leave. We have the other residents to think about." His elegant fingers trembled a little as he reached for the water glass. The shadows under his eyes hinted of a lousy night's sleep. I imagined how Geoff was feeling after nineteen years of living with my sister. I recalled the letter from L'Abri to Dr. Byrne that had been safely tucked away in my filing cabinet seven years earlier. The grievances were nothing new at the time, but recorded on paper, they had made my head spin: flaking out for hours, swinging into hyper mode, talking continually with disjointed thoughts, disrupting conversations, drinking copious amounts of water, obsessively throwing things out. Nancy was not easy to live with.

"Where will she go?" I asked in a small voice.

"Your father left her a trust. Perhaps you could set Nancy up in her own place."

He gestured towards the window. Beyond the pretty geraniums loomed a high-rise tower in a sad stage of decline. The concrete walls were pitted with age and streaked with rust.

"Live on her own?"

"Perhaps it'd be better that way."

"Who would pay the bills? Who would keep an eye on her?"

The director and I both knew how that story would unfold.

"I'm sure you'll figure something out," he said.

"When does she have to leave?"

"Immediately, I'm afraid."

"You're aware I'm leaving for Costa Rica in early January?"

"We were hoping you would move her belongings before you go. We need to find another roommate for the apartment."

Fuelled by sudden rage, I scraped the chair away from the director, his vintage oak desk, the thick dog-eared file and stood up to regain control. The height of the desk hid my wobbling knees. My brain whirled, desperate to find an escape route. Delaying our departure was unacceptable.

"I'll pay three months' rent to keep the belongings in her room."

The director shook his head.

"We only hold rooms for residents in the event of a relapse."

I glared at him.

"Is this not a relapse?"

He hesitated. I had him.

"Okay, ninety days. For her belongings."

The negotiations were over, not that anything had been negotiated. The director handed me a white envelope. Expulsion papers.

The empty waiting room at the External Clinic for Psychotic Disorders gave the impression that mental illness was on holiday like everyone else, my sister and I being the exception. Lights were dimmed and office doors were closed. The television screen attached to the wall was pitch black and the sharp smell of disinfectant was noticeably absent. Nancy's legs swung back and forth under the waiting room chair, like a child awaiting punishment. I touched the back of her arm.

"You've done nothing wrong," I said with affection.

She yanked her arm from my hand.

"I know that!" she belted out in a baritone voice.

The injustice stung.

"I was just trying to help."

"I'm the victim."

"The director told me that you spat at Geoff."

I knew it was a mistake, but the damage was already done.

"I DID NOT!"

"Why would he make that up?"

"LIES. ALL LIES!"

She stormed into the bathroom, leaving the door slightly ajar. Running water gushed into the sink and her hands pounded the paper towel dispenser. She ripped off a sheet, then another and another, the tap still turned on full blast. My sister's illness was too solipsistic for her to worry about climate change.

We followed Dr. Byrne down the hall into his office. He opened the white envelope and read the letter I had paraphrased over the phone.

"Not to worry. You can stay on a ward in the Burgess Pavilion until we find you a place to live."

Nancy bolted to her feet. The force of her body came close to overturning the solid wood visitor chair.

"Being in the Douglas is going backwards!" she cried.

Dr. Byrne remained seated.

"I assure you. This is temporary. You'll be free to come and go during the day," he said calmly.

She lowered into her chair, defeated. "Free?"

"Yes."

"How long?"

"A few weeks."

"Can I still go to weaving?"

"Absolutely. But first, we need to have you admitted. I'll call emergency to let them know you're coming."

"What about my clothes? A toothbrush?"

"I'm sure your sister will help you out."

The light in the office dimmed. Flying snow scratched at the window. Dr. Byrne switched on his desk lamp and reached for the phone to make the necessary arrangements. Nancy and I thanked him and filed out of the office.

The tires crunched on the fresh fallen snow as I steered out of the clinic towards the main entrance of the Douglas Hospital. We turned a sharp left at the gate. The Perry Pavilion loomed before us.

"You're lucky to be getting away from all of this," she muttered, and then told me to drive straight, turn right, turn left. I parked in the lot next to the emergency. We shuffled to the door where the attendant at the security desk asked for our coats, bags and my belt. A precaution, he said, and then motioned us towards a windowless waiting room that made the External Clinic for Psychotic Disorders look like a hotel lobby.

"Hello," Nancy shouted at a hooded man on the far side of the room.

"Shhhh. Not the place for chit-chat," I whispered.

The hooded man stared at us with feral eyes. Even Nancy looked away.

"How am I supposed to keep in touch while you're in Puerto Rico?" she asked.

"You mean Costa Rica."

"Puerto Rica, Puerto Costa, Rico Rica. Whatever."

"You can call me on my cell. It's a local call from Montreal."

"How can I call you without a phone?"

Good question. Stuck in hospital, she wouldn't have access to her landline. I sighed.

"Too bad you don't want to use the iPad. We could Skype or FaceTime."

"I shake too much to use your gadgets."

"If you focus and relax, maybe your fingers won't shake as much."

"Easy for you to say."

"I'm sure the staff will let you use the phone at the nursing station. I'll call you every day, okay?"

Silence.

"Dr. Byrne seemed pretty sure of finding you a place to live."

More silence. I leaned in a little closer.

"I'm so sorry this has happened, darling," I said softly.

"Enjoy your vacation in Costa Rica."

A male attendant approached us. He was gentle and nice-looking. Nancy left willingly, without saying goodbye. The waiting room blurred.

"Are you okay?"

The man with feral eyes was standing three feet away. He offered me a tissue from his pocket-size Kleenex pack. Too choked to speak, I accepted the gift with a nod and turned towards the security desk to retrieve my belongings. I hurried out to the parking lot, the belt and bag in my hand, my coat unzipped, and proceeded to scrape off the thin layer of ice on the windshield. My frozen fingers gripped the steering wheel as I drove through the hospital gate with the defroster on high. My sister's nineteen-year hiatus was over. Her future looked grim. Another hospitalization. More shitty group homes. I reached for the tissue, a sweet gesture from a caring stranger. I didn't deserve such kindness. I was abandoning her, just as our parents had done.

My knuckle made a bizarre clicking noise when the doctor forced my third finger to bend. He diagnosed my condition as "stenosing tenosynovitis" or trigger finger. Nothing urgent, he said, although the joint might become stuck in a closed position. He referred me to a specialist, Dr. Navi, coincidentally the owner of the dock my father had once swum to.

"How are your parents?" asked Dr. Navi, looking up from my file.

"They passed seven years ago."

It felt like another lifetime. It felt like yesterday.

"My deepest sympathies. Your father loved to swim in the lake, didn't he?"

I cringed from the childhood memory of the Navi's enthusiastic golden lab jumping on my father during his afternoon ritual swim. My father panicked and began to sink under the eighty-pound weight. Fortunately, Nancy was paying close attention. She dove in, swam out to our father, grabbed his arm and pushed the dog away. Later that evening, my father discovered a bottle of Brunello di Montalcino on his doorstep and an apologetic note from the neighbours. He asked Nancy to return the wine. Our parents remained furious about the dog incident for years and retold the tale many times. Thinking back, the larger and far more interesting story was how Nancy had managed to pull our father free.

"Your sister, how's she?" asked Dr. Navi.

"Up and down," I replied, my standard response.

"I remember the time she came to our house . . ."

I braced myself to hear about the bottle of returned wine and the rejected apology. My parents' former neighbour proceeded to tell a very different story. My sister had knocked on his door asking for help. Our father was unwell and needed medical attention. Dr. Navi rushed over with his doctor's bag. When he arrived, our mother was hysterical and our father was shaking under a pile of blankets with a mild case of hypothermia from the lake. He had insisted on swimming in late September. "Nancy was the calm one," the doctor said. "She had her act together."

I thanked Dr. Navi and tucked the cortisone prescription he had written into my wallet. His story about my sister followed me out of the examination room, through the clinic and onto the street. I hesitated on the sidewalk, blinking at the late January afternoon sky that was strangely dazzling despite the grey sweep of cirrus clouds. In the face of emergency, Nancy had acted sanely with a cooler head than our parents. I removed my sunglasses from the case and headed towards home, my stiff and angry finger completely forgotten.

22

JANUARY 2016, THE AIRPORT TAXI turned onto the dirt road and pulled up to our iron gate. The hand-painted sign for Casa Verano was lying face down on the ground, half-eaten by termites. We took turns struggling with the rusted lock. A hard whack from a stone finally turned the key. "Watch out," Keith shouted. The stone walkway was coated in green slime, a slippery hazard of Costa Rica's rainy season. We dragged the luggage to the front porch, our foreheads dripping with sweat. I unzipped my carry-on, pulled out a sundress and flip-flops and slumped into the worn leather rocking chair that had survived another year.

"Aren't you going in?" Keith asked, jingling the front door keys.

"I'm in no rush. It's gonna be hotter than hell in there."

Keith returned a few minutes later in a T-shirt and bathing trunks.

"You were right," he said. "The house is an oven! It'll cool down with the windows open and the fans on. Let's head to the beach."

I pushed up to standing. My legs were already wobbly from the heat. The beach would be cooler with the breeze from the ocean.

"You go ahead. I'll catch up. I have a couple of things to do."

He hesitated like he might ask me what was so important that I couldn't just leave.

"Okay, but don't take too long. Sunset is coming."

The gate creaked open and clanged shut. I changed into the sundress and meandered over to the small pool. Reptilian beady eyes peered at me through the weave of hibiscus, a member of the extended iguana family that lived on our roof. I called them all Iggy. He sneezed at me, as iguanas do, and bit off one of the few remaining flowers. Last winter, the gardener had suggested warding Iggy off with pesticides, but the town was already full of toxins from machines that sprayed ditches for dengue, from wood-burning fires and from septic pipes that emptied into the ocean. I settled on the cement edge of the pool and splashed my feet in the cool water, oblivious to the microscopic ants scurrying around me. Ten seconds later, I bolted to standing and ran to the outdoor shower. The stings from the invisible ants felt like shards of glass, punishment for procrastinating about making the phone call.

The nurse who answered was new to the Burgess Pavilion; she had no idea who my sister was. Call back in fifteen minutes, she suggested. On my second attempt, I was informed that Nancy was at the pharmacy in Verdun and due back in thirty minutes. I wandered back to the pool in my flip-flops with the phone in my hand, mindful to avoid the cement edge. At four o'clock, my third call, the nurse placed me on hold; my sister was in the bathroom. I closed my eyes and rocked back and forth on the front porch.

"Hello?" Her voice sounded tenuous, far away.

"Hi, darling."

"Phew, it's you. Are you there?"

"Yup. Arrived about an hour ago."

"Did you go in the pool?"

"Not really." I rubbed my thigh, still sensitive from the stings.

"Not really sounds like yes."

"You're hard to get hold of," I said, ignoring her comment.

"I was out."

"That's great that you're allowed to come and go."

"It depends on the staff. Some of the nurses don't believe me. They don't bother to check the notes in my file."

"That's horrible. Should I call the unit coordinator?"

"It won't do much good. Who's groaning in the background?"

I scanned the jungle looking for the familiar black shape swinging from tree to tree.

"It's a howler monkey. He'll be gone soon."

"Sounds like the guy in the room across the hall. He's doing it now. Listen."

I pressed the phone into my ear. She was right. The throaty roar was similar.

"What's his story?" I asked.

"Delusional and paranoid. We don't get along."

"Does he do this all the time?"

"You get used to the noise."

My mind wandered back to childhood, to my quiet sister. Did the illness make her immune to loud outbursts, including her own? Or were there other reasons? I pictured her being forced to endure group therapy at the Allan Memorial, the lone adolescent in a circle of sick adults. The therapist opens her arms and asks the group to express themselves. The patient across from Nancy stands up. "Why am I here?" he asks. He repeats the question over and over like a mantra, gaining volume each time. Someone in the circle yells, "Shut up!" and the man raises his voice even louder. Nancy can't think straight with all the noise; it's hard enough with all those pills inside her. She opens her mouth and releases a shrill teenage scream. Faces turn. Her numb lips melt into a small smile from her new discovery—the power of her vocal cords. Her family will be stunned by the new voice. If they disapprove, she will outshout them. The range of her repertoire will free her.

"Have you made any friends on the ward?" I asked.

Nancy snorted.

"Are you kidding? I bet you and Keith have tons of friends in Costa Costa."

"Costa Costa. That's hilarious, darling. And you're right, it's more expensive than we thought."

"When do I get to visit?"

"I've told you before. You wouldn't like the heat."

"I could get used to it. And you have a pool."

"The sidewalks are broken. The surf is wild. There's not much to do. You'd get bored quickly."

"*You're* not bored."

"I write. I read. I go to yoga class. You don't do those things."

"You don't want me there."

"It's not practical."

"Is buying a house in Central America practical?"

"It's a break for me. I need it."

"You need a break? I need a break!"

A catfight broke out on the other side of the cement wall. A local ginger tabby named Don Carlos bounded into our garden and onto the front porch. I flattened the fur on his spine and squeezed his spiked tail back to normal size. No visible scratches; he had escaped his attacker, an option that was not available to me.

"Any news on a group home?" I asked.

"Nothing."

"I'll call the social worker tomorrow."

"Can you call now?"

A blood-orange glow flickered through the trees. I was missing the sunset.

"It's too late to call."

"I need you to call now."

"Tomorrow morning."

"*First thing* tomorrow!"

"Yes, first thing."

"We'll speak tomorrow, too?"

"Yes. Every day."

"Promise?"

Promise to my mother, promise to my sister.

We hung up, the first call completed; eighty-nine more calls to go. I considered the efficiency of her flying down for a week. I would save hours of telephone time. But she would trip over the rickety sidewalks and despise the young girls on the beach with their G-string bikinis and sun salutations. The snakes and the scorpions—anything that would bite and sting— would be drawn to my sister. We would be stuck in paradise with her demands and bitter complaints. My throat would constrict like it did after our last trip. London calling all over again.

I locked the front door and hurried towards the gate, avoiding the slippery stones on the walkway. So close to the equator, Costa Rica in daylight follows a rigid schedule of twelve hours, plus or minus thirty minutes, depending on the time of year, a phenomenon that disappoints northerners who expect the warm light to linger into the evening. Instead, dusk is fleeting; the sun falls like a lead lure into the ocean or, in the case of the view from Casa Verano, into the jungle. A few feet from where I stood at the gate with my key, a pauraque flew up from the undergrowth and glided in and out of the shadows between the guanacaste trees. The wings caught a flash of dying light as the bird lifted to join the other pauraques in their erratic bat-like flight over our house. They called to each other in long slurred whistles. Purr-WHEE-eer. Purr-WHEE-eer.

The nocturnal song followed me out of the gate and down the dirt road. An old dread returned to my chest, the same sinking sensation as when the screeching nighthawks circled my parents' house and I pulled the cover over my head to protect me from the screams coming from my sister's room. I remembered the words of expat George from last winter: *You can run away to the tropics with just a carry-on, but sooner or later the rest of your baggage shows up.* My pura vida dream was falling fast, in sync with the setting sun.

I pulled off my winter gloves, squeezed the steering wheel with both hands and smiled. The cortisone prescribed by Dr. Navi was working on my third finger, a good omen for the afternoon. The mild winter temperature was another positive sign, although I was wary; winter in Montreal was far from over in early February. At precisely five minutes before one o'clock p.m., I turned onto Benny and double-parked in front of my sister's building. She was waiting on the edge of the sidewalk, shopping bag in hand.

"I need to put my things in the back of the car," she said.

"No problem."

I stepped out to help her, determined to make a success of our outing.

"You were on time," Nancy said, handing me her bag.

"I'm a couple of minutes early. A rare event!"

She didn't respond, a minor victory on my part.

"I'd like to know more about this therapist we're going to see," Nancy asked.

My esthetician had told me about Lucia while prodding my chin with small jolts of electrical current. I didn't dare tell Nancy that Lucia was a shamanic practitioner. The possibility that an entity from the spirit world was responsible for my sister's schizoaffective mood disorder seemed worthy of exploration. Nancy, however, was much too practical to embrace that which she could not see.

"Lucia is an energetic healer."

"Hmm. Sounds like a waste of money. Is this going to cost as much as the last one?"

I hadn't bothered to ask Lucia how much she charged. At least $120, I assumed. My sister was skeptical. She maintains that psychiatrists and psychologists often struggle with their own mental health maladies;

many people would agree with her, including myself. Convincing her to see a psychotherapist was no easy feat. Finding one who accepted clients with a chronic mental illness was another hurdle. They want "the easy ones," according to my sister.

In the year prior to our meeting with Lucia, I'd convinced Nancy to try out two different therapists my research had uncovered with the hope that the sessions might help alleviate her anxiety and reduce the frequency of her outbursts. The first therapist, a former nurse, suggested that my sister's condition was triggered by sexual trauma, a theory Nancy found ludicrous. The second therapist had worked at the Douglas Hospital and knew all about the side room on Perry 2C—a perfect fit for my sister. Nancy quit after four sessions. She told me that psychotherapy was demeaning and made her feel stigmatized, a response I'd never considered. Had she been telling me this all along and I wasn't listening? I had been too focused on what would work for me, even though I wasn't acting on it, a textbook case of projection, my sister would say. Once again, she would be right.

We turned onto a quiet street that curved into a residential development. The mid-century bungalows brought back pleasant memories. Under the two-foot layer of snow, I pictured well-tended lawns and flower gardens. Nancy, who rarely paid attention to landscape, was staring out the window.

"What ya thinking, Nance?"

She hesitated. I braced myself for another question about Lucia.

"This reminds me of Tettenhall Road in Etobicoke," she said.

I reached over and patted her mittened hand. Our minds were aligned for once, another good omen. Taking my sister to Lucia was not demeaning nor would she feel stigmatized. What if there was an entity haunting her? A little far-fetched perhaps, but no stone unturned. It was the right thing to do. I pulled up to the address Lucia had given me, a two-storey beige-brick house. We had arrived ten minutes early. Nancy, unable to wait, marched up the flagstone path and pressed the bell. The door opened almost immediately.

Lucia was dressed casually like us, in leggings and a loose sweater, her long dark hair pulled back. She invited us into a bright kitchen that smelled like freshly brewed coffee and something sweet. Nancy accepted the kind offer of tea and asked a multitude of questions while we waited for the water to boil. Lucia responded to each inquiry with patience:

she was forty-two, married twice, had two daughters, was born in El Salvador. Her calm voice was soothing, like water running over river stones. I leaned against the kitchen wall and observed; this was Nancy's appointment, not mine.

Lucia led us down a narrow stairwell to her basement office, a small carpeted room with a window looking up to the street. The walls were covered in woodcarvings and woven textiles like the handicrafts we'd hung at Casa Verano. Nancy settled in an armchair. I sat on the sofa.

"Are you comfortable?" Lucia asked my sister.

Nancy pointed at me.

"I'd rather be on the sofa."

I stood and offered Nancy my place, our little dance. She stayed seated.

"It's not so bad here, I guess."

I gritted my teeth. More than forty minutes had passed since we'd arrived. Would we run out of time?

"Why are you here?" Lucia asked Nancy.

"Because my sister wants me to talk to you."

"What about you? Do you want to talk to me?"

"I'm not sure."

"That's okay. We don't have to talk."

Nancy studied the books on the shelves above Lucia's desk.

"Do you read the bible?" Nancy asked. Her gaze was fixed on a worn spine that had also caught my attention.

"I read lots of books. You?"

"I mostly listen to the radio. My sister's the literary one."

The comment felt loaded and tipped my mood which had been wavering since the interrogation in the kitchen. I steadied myself with the reminder that the illness had diminished Nancy's cognitive skills. She could only focus on a few paragraphs at a time. Yet, her mind had remained razor sharp. She didn't miss a beat.

"What kind of therapist are you?" Nancy asked. It was a reasonable question.

Lucia smiled. "I don't consider myself a therapist. I'm more of a guide. I'm happy to show you if you'd like."

Nancy remained stone-faced, possibly confounded. If this wasn't psychotherapy, what was it?

Lucia lifted a small rattle. The head was covered in animal skin, the handle made of carved wood.

"Would you give me permission to use this?"

"Our parents had a rattle. A gourd filled with coffee beans they brought back from the Caribbean."

"Not quite the same thing. May I use it? I need your permission."

Nancy shrugged. "Why not?"

The hiss of the rattling filled the small basement room. My sister's comments, should she have any, were unheard. A beating drum from Lucia's iPhone joined in. I unfolded my arms and uncrossed my legs. The low percussive tone steadied my heart and grounded my feet. My eyes started to close. Deep in the jungle, the blade of my machete sliced through the thick brush and exposed an ancient tree in the middle of the path. The trunk was at least six feet in diameter. I reached for a low branch and pulled myself up. A spiral wedge was carved twelve inches into the bark, more than enough to accommodate my feet. I climbed the makeshift staircase higher and higher around the ancient tree. Finally, I could see blue sky. Another two or three turns and I would reach the top.

The drumbeat slowed. The rattling stopped. My jungle vision cleared. Lucia's eyes were shining.

"How do you feel?" she asked my sister.

"I'm thirsty," Nancy replied.

Lucia poured from the water pitcher on her table.

"Would you like to know what I saw?" she asked, handing Nancy the glass.

"Sure."

"A baby elephant."

Nancy screwed up her face. "An *elephant*?"

"Elephants are strong and powerful beings," I said quickly.

Lucia continued.

"The baby elephant is curious about the world, so she wanders off the path. Her parents nudge her back, gently. She wanders off again, a little further. This is what she does. She wanders. But she always finds her way back."

Nancy checked her watch and I glanced at the clock on the bookshelf. We'd been sitting in the room for over an hour. How did that happen?

"How much do I owe you?" Nancy asked.

Lucia hesitated.

"How about forty-five dollars?"

With a quavering hand, Nancy wrote a cheque and then turned to me.

"Can we go for coffee?"

I sighed inwardly, annoyed at myself for wasting everyone's time. I should have known better. Still, I had enjoyed my jungle vision, whatever it meant.

Lucia pulled me back on our way out the front door. Her hand felt warm on my arm.

"Call me when you get home," she whispered.

I called two hours later from my hammock chair. Lucia explained she couldn't do much. Nancy was too frightened to open up to the spirit world, worried that people would call her crazy and lock her up. I had never thought about that.

"There's something else I wanted to tell you."

"What's that?" I asked.

"It is not up to you to bring your sister back to the path. She will return on her own. All you have to do is give her the confidence to find her way. She is going to be okay. Life always brings her back. You are not responsible for her. You're free to play."

The hammock chair rocked in a clockwise rotation, a new view with each swing: my grandmother's portrait; my mother's portrait; photographs of my children; the bay window and the honey locust in the front yard that we planted twenty-seven years ago and was now as tall as the house; the peeling paint on the radiator; the to-do list on the whiteboard; and, finally, an abstract painting Nancy had titled "My Sister" hanging over our father's campaign desk. She had told me I was the subject. The woman's eyes were emerald green and Picassoesque, large and almond-shaped, lines swirling with energy, a strong gaze.

I pushed out of the hammock chair, grabbed a marker and wrote *My sister is not my responsibility* on the whiteboard. Underneath, in smaller letters, I added *Feel free to play*. I read the ten words out loud. My voice faded on the second repetition. Easy to say. How to put into practice? I turned away, totally baffled.

23

APRIL 5, 2016, THE EVE OF OUR DEPARTURE from Costa Rica, Keith and I reached the observation deck at the Parque Nacional Volcán Poás. On the same afternoon, my sister was transferred from the Burgess Pavilion to Levinschi House, a transition home on the grounds of the Douglas Hospital. We had driven five hours on winding Costa Rican roads; Nancy had travelled two minutes. Thin wisps of steam rose from the fumaroles 9,000 feet above sea level. Poás had flared up thirty-nine times since 1828, and experts claimed another blast was due. The stench of rotten eggs and a massive crater bubbling with liquid sulphur didn't faze me, nor did the evacuation signs in case of emergency. The more pressing concern was my sister's next eruption.

Two days later, in the midst of moving Nancy's belongings from the apartment at L'Abri, my presence was requested at Levinschi House. I spotted Nancy a block away. She was guarding a vacant spot between two parked cars on boulevard LaSalle, a burning cigarette pressed between her lips. Following our parents' death, Nancy often bummed smokes, an excuse to strike up conversation. That afternoon, she was alone, puffing like mad. I backed into the vacant spot, unbuckled and greeted her on the sidewalk. We'd spoken daily during our three-month separation; a kiss or a hug did not feel warranted. I gestured at the pack of du Mauriers in her right hand.

"I hope that hasn't become a habit."

She surveyed me up and down and then flicked the burning cigarette onto the spring grass.

"I joined a quit-smoking group while you were away."

"Great! How's that working?"

Her closed-mouth smile warned me to prepare.

"I learned how to smoke better."

I rolled my eyes, but said nothing. Better that way.

"You've had too much sun," she said.

I inspected my freckled hands. "We spent most of the time on our porch. The beach was too hot. Hotter than last year."

"That doesn't make any sense. Why bother going?"

I shrugged.

"Did you use sunscreen?

"Of course."

"Doesn't look like it."

A cluster of millennials were gathered in front of Levinschi House. At sixty-two, Nancy revolved in a different world from the younger residents. The elder status allowed her to wiggle out of group therapy and substance abuse counselling. She had full control of her time, which she spent alone or on the phone with me, Julie, my children, L'Atelier staff and former roommate Geoff even though they had parted under tense circumstances. Nancy's telephone contacts were constantly expanding.

The millennials parted as I followed my sister up the front steps. She pressed on the bell and turned to her audience, me included.

"Levinschi House doesn't look like a prison, but it is."

The door buzzed open. Nancy reported to reception for the obligatory check-in. A young woman looked up at us. *Claire* was printed on the name tag hanging from her neck. I recognized her from Nancy's description: bright and bouncy with bovine brown eyes.

"This is my sister. The one who lives in Costa Rica."

"Good for her," said Claire.

I cleared my throat. "For the record, I live in Montreal most of the year."

"But you have a house in Costa Rica," Nancy said, a sharpness in her voice. "And a pool."

Claire smiled. "If I had a *casa* in Costa Rica, I'd move there full-time."

I poked Nancy with my elbow. "See, darling, it could be worse. I could be living in Costa Rica year-round!"

Claire laughed. She likely had heard more than one story about me. Nancy glowered at us. I had one-upped her and was chumming up to a staff member she was envious of. Two infractions. Nancy grabbed my arm.

"Come see my suite."

We climbed a staircase to the second floor and navigated down a narrow hallway reminiscent of a budget-priced hotel in lower Manhattan. Nancy stopped at the last door on the left.

"Voilà!" she cried, stepping into the room.

The reference to a prison was not far off. My sister's single bed was pushed tight against the wall to accommodate a bedside table and allow access to a small square window. I raised the blind and peered through dirty glass at boulevard LaSalle.

"Hey, you can see a bit of river from here."

"Never bothered looking."

On hands and knees, she pulled a suitcase from under the bed.

"This is my clothes dresser."

I giggled to keep things light. "Not exactly the Ritz, huh?"

"Not exactly."

Retracing our steps along the hall and down the stairs, we arrived at a dimly lit dining area. Nancy pointed to a single chair and table in a dark corner of the room. Her table. The institutional setting reminded me of the cafeteria at Westmount High, where my friends had shielded me from my crazy sister. I had acted like a spoiled brat, just like the kids who'd made fun of her. No amount of caring could change the past.

Claire tapped my shoulder. The staff meeting was about to begin. She led me up a different staircase from the one Nancy and I had taken minutes earlier. We navigated down another narrow hallway. Levinschi House was surprisingly complex for its compact size. Claire hesitated in front of an open door. The staff lounge.

"Come with me," she said to Nancy. "We can hang out in the office."

My sister's cheeks turned crimson and her eyes opened wide, then her face disappeared as Claire pulled her away and someone closed the door. I chose a seat next to the window, the farthest point from the kerfuffle happening in the hallway. I could have spoken up. I could have requested my sister's presence in the staff lounge. Instead, I ignored the stinging unfairness and settled in my seat, relieved that the meeting would proceed without interruption.

The house psychiatrist, Dr. Ford, introduced himself and five other staff members. He looked like he had sounded over the phone: thin, fragile, close to retirement. My heart sank with his opening statement: "We can't keep Nancy here much longer." This was the same refrain I'd heard during our long-distance call two weeks earlier. They still hadn't figured out what to do with her. I questioned the value of my two-page document I was handing out to the doctor, the social worker, the two nurses and two attendants: four discussion points and a list of living options. Papers rustled as the staff reviewed my notes. The social worker sitting beside me was the first to speak.

"There's still an opening at the group home on Park Row in Notre-Dame-de-Grâce."

I wanted to scream. Could the social worker not read? *Point 1: Dr. Byrne expresses concern that a group home would threaten Nancy's autonomy. Point 2: Nancy is not a team player; she sets her own rules.*

"Nancy would have problems in a group home," I said evenly.

"What kind of problems?"

"She ended up at the Douglas because she didn't get along with her roommates."

"She seems fine here."

Did the staff not know my sister? Had her free and easy schedule allowed her to slip through the cracks?

"No outbursts? No clashes with the residents?" I asked the room.

The social worker shrugged.

"Nothing stands out."

The other staff nodded in agreement, except for Dr. Ford who was reviewing the second page of my document.

"Do you have any suggestions?" he asked, looking up.

What he really meant was "We have no clue what to do with your sister." The meeting slipped into an uncomfortable silence. We were at a standstill.

Four months earlier, the director of L'Abri en Ville had pointed out that Nancy's trust fund would cover the expenses of an apartment. My sister's insistent knocking on the staff lounge door reminded me why I had rejected his suggestion so vehemently. The additional responsibility was terrifying. I returned to the document to steady myself. *Point 3: Nancy does well with a structured schedule. Point 4: Nancy needs ongoing support and should not be isolated.* My fingers gripped the paper. I resolved to hold off proposing the last-resort option noted at the bottom of page two until all others had been eliminated. Surely the staff had ideas.

I scanned their faces. All blank except for the doctor who was watching me, reading my mind perhaps.

The knocking stopped. Claire must have called for reinforcements to drag Nancy away. My poor sister, banned from a meeting about *her* life. What kind of godforsaken place would she live in next? Another prison . . . or worse? Nancy was right when she said I had too much sun. I was swimming in abundance compared to her. Why couldn't she have a taste of normality?

I closed my eyes to recall the wording in my father's will: *The trustee will use the funds at her discretion to provide comfort for Nancy.* Or something like that. My firmness wavered, then dissolved in an instant like salt in warm water. I shifted to the edge of the chair and dove in.

"If I were to move Nancy into her own apartment, what support would the health-care system provide?"

The silence in the room shifted to surprise. Or was it relief? Again, the social worker was the first to speak, the conduit between Levinschi House and the outside world.

"She would be eligible for weekly home visits arranged by the closest CLSC clinic."

Once a week didn't sound like much.

"How soon would the visits start?"

"Your sister would be on a waiting list."

I knew about wait lists. Nancy wasn't going anywhere anytime soon.

"How long will we have to wait?"

"A month. Maybe two."

"By July 1?"

"Yes."

"Can she stay here until then?"

The social worker glanced at the doctor, who nodded.

"Yes," she said. "We can make an exception."

"All right then."

Handshakes sealed the deal, the conclusion of another sister negotiation. I left the staff lounge on shaky feet, distressed by the daunting responsibility that lay ahead. Claire waved goodbye from her desk at reception. I didn't bother to ask about my sister's whereabouts. Wherever she was, the good news would spread soon enough. I navigated around the millennials on the front steps.

"Do you think it's a prison?" one of them asked.

I turned and faced the small crowd. The young faces were fresh despite their ailments. They made mine feel worn and old. I forced a small smile.

"There are many kinds of prisons," I said.

The social worker from Burgess Pavilion called as I pulled away from the sidewalk. I double parked on boulevard LaSalle with my four-ways flashing. She'd just heard about the staff meeting from her colleague at Levinschi House, how I had offered to set Nancy up in her own home.

"The staff seems to think she'll be fine," I told her.

"And what do you think?" she asked.

"She'll love it. No rules!"

"Exactly. Which is why she wouldn't last in a group home."

"You understand!"

"Levinschi House doesn't know your sister like we do. Look, I'm no longer working on the file, but I know how involved you are. May I be frank?"

"Please."

"You're not doing Nancy any favours by enabling her. If you continue to let her get away with belligerent behaviour, she'll end up alone in long-term care. Do you understand what I mean, how you're not helping her?"

I understood perfectly; later I would understand differently. I veered back onto boulevard LaSalle and accelerated, my eyes stinging from the unfair criticism. How dare she accuse me of enabling my sister! I was kind and generous, a saint, albeit an unwilling one. The social worker had no clue what my life was like or what my sister had been through. We both deserved sympathy. My foot pressed hard on the gas, fuelled by indignation. I slammed on the brakes just in time at the pedestrian crossing. Two middle-aged women in matching spring jackets and leather boots crossed the street, their arms linked. Sisters. The older one tapped the hood of my car and pointed at the white-painted line my front tires had crossed. I lowered the window to apologize, but the impatient driver behind me blasted his horn. The sisters would never know I was a good person with good intentions.

I pushed the social worker's words aside for later contemplation. More pressing matters required my attention. I needed to find an apartment with a convenient location, walking distance from shops and from me. After thirty years, my sister would have her own bathroom and a kitchen. She could invite me over for lunch, and afterwards, we could drop in at a neighbourhood café buzzing with friendly staff and patrons. The rich aroma of coffee beans and cinnamon buns would greet us. We'd sip on lattes and catch up on each other's life, raising our voices to be heard over the roar of the espresso machine, laughing like old friends. The fantasy circled me with comforting arms. I drove home in a bubble of calm, unaware that my four-way flashers were still blinking.

That night I woke gasping for air under the blanket. Had I made a huge mistake? Was I an enabler? I pictured my sister's prison-cell room, the narrow cot tight to the wall, clothes stashed under the bed, the dirty window. The image soothed my panic. I'd done the right thing.

We settled in the rear of a river raft on a two-seater bench tied to bamboo pontoons with twine. Our captain, in low-hanging shorts, poled through reflections of fluffy clouds and mango trees weighted by vines. I glanced sideways at Keith, grateful for his suggestion to book a last-minute sun holiday in February, one that had brought us closer together. I was free to play, just as Lucia had said. Shamans and baby elephants had been pushed far into the background. Our captain steered down the Rio Grande towards a sandbar and the raft slid onto land. The air was still and sticky. I wiggled out of my shorts into a bathing suit under the privacy of a sarong. The fresh water was cool, without the ocean's stinging salt or dangerous undertow. I swam towards the middle of the river, kicking in a jerky circular motion, hands and feet unsynchronized, head above water. My crawl was still amateurish, but the years had granted me endurance. Keith swam towards me, grinning. I knew what he saw. His partner was beaming with happiness.

The waterproof, zippered pouch on the raft chimed with crystal bells from an incoming call, the custom ringtone my son had suggested for his aunt's number. I hesitated, treading water next to Keith. He was watching me closely, his eyes sparkling with river turquoise. Five rings, six, seven, eight. The chiming stopped. We climbed back onto the bamboo pontoons and resettled on the platform, drying ourselves with my sarong. Our captain pushed off the sandbar to continue the journey downstream. Around a sharp bend, the river narrowed and the raft picked up speed. The chiming bells started up again. My chest tightened from the unwarranted intrusion. I let go of Keith's hand and unzipped the pouch. "You don't have to answer," he said. "She'll call back." Five rings, six. Keith was right. She would call back. Seven rings, eight. I grabbed the phone.

"Hi, Nance, I can't really talk now."

"Finally! Where were you? I've been calling all morning!"

My sister's shrill voice trumpeted across the Rio Grande, the call of the baby elephant. The bamboo pontoons under the raft knocked against the water as we bounced over small rapids.

I tightened my grip on the phone and glanced at our captain. His pants had fallen even lower over his hips. If my sister had an iPhone, I could share the view. She may not care about me, but she would be interested in him.

"Not a good time for me. I'll call you back."

"Not a good time for me either! Freezing rain today. I'm afraid to leave the condo."

I hated her. I hated myself for answering.

"I need you to make a call for me," she said.

The pharmacist had made a mistake with her Dispill blister pack and some pills were missing. She had tried to fix the problem over the phone and had been ignored. The staff didn't take her seriously. They had blown her off. She needed me to contact the pharmacist as soon as possible.

"I'll call the pharmacy later. I have to go now," I said quietly.

The raft slowed and the river widened. My sister continued to talk. When was I going to call the pharmacy? She needed the problem solved now. And there was a second problem she needed to discuss. I hung up without saying goodbye.

The emerald valley dulled to grey. Passing scenery blurred. I no longer heard the crunching in the gravel riverbed from the captain's pole or the sweet birdsong in the mango branches. The lemony scent of the blossoms on a passing bush was lost on me. My mind was in my home office, reading Lucia's words on the whiteboard.

24

NANCY AND I ATTENDED A DISCHARGE MEETING in the staff lounge on the eve of her checkout from Levinschi House. The procedure was uneventful, a formality. We were almost done when Dr. Ford expressed a last-minute concern.

"Will she be safe living on her own?" he asked. "What if she slips in the shower?"

Nancy shot out of her chair.

"I'm sixty-two years old, Dr. Ford. You are what? Sixty-five? Are you afraid of slipping in the shower?"

I refrained from snickering until we were on the sidewalk.

"You set that doctor straight, girl!" I told my sister, patting her back.

"Someone had to," she replied in a deadpan voice.

"Why would he question the decision at the last minute? Not very professional!"

She shrugged.

"He's probably on meds."

I explained to the rental agent that Nancy suffered from mood swings. He was more concerned about the non-existent credit rating than her mental health. The application was accepted on the condition that we both sign the lease. On the first day of July 2016, Nancy moved into a one-bedroom unit on the second floor of a low-rise, LEED-certified condo complex on avenue Benny in central Notre-Dame-de-Grâce, a perfect location for her. The condo was spacious and equipped with brand-new stainless-steel appliances. Nancy would be free to wash her clothes as often as she desired, a compulsion of hers that had caused problems in the past. A balcony off the living area looked onto leafy maples and the perennial gardens of the single-family homes across the street. The grocery store, pharmacy, CLSC medical clinic and Benny pool were within a two-block radius. I'd furnished the condo with our parents' rattan sofa and chairs, side tables, linen, kitchenware and artwork that had cluttered my basement for three-and-a-half years. A new television and double bed were unwrapped, ready for use. The kitchen cupboards were scrubbed down and filled with supplies, the floor swept and mopped. I looked forward to my sister's reaction to her new perfect home—and to our sleepover. A celebration!

"So, what do you think?" I asked.

She frowned at the exposed cement ceiling.

"Needs painting."

I laughed.

"That's deliberate. The industrial look is trending."

"The industrial look needs painting. This is not a factory."

I sashayed to the middle of the room and spread my arms wide à la Vanna White.

"What do you think of the furniture?"

She lowered onto the rattan sofa facing our mother's three-by-four-foot painting of our parents' Laurentian cottage. The wooden frame creaked under her.

"Ancient, like me," she said.

I gestured at the two-person teak table.

"I bought this for you. An early birthday gift."

"Is it sturdy?" she asked, eyeing the mid-century-style legs.

I shook the table. She was right, the legs were a little wobbly.

"You can always exchange it—"

"I'd rather exchange Mom's painting."

"I thought the cottage would trigger good memories. You loved going there."

"Not her best work."

Undefeated, I picked up the remote and pressed the menu button. Nancy rarely watched television when she lived in the apartment at L'Abri. Being alone might change that.

"Check out the Super Package, tons of channels."

"You know, I don't know how to use those gizmos," she said.

At six that evening we ate the pasta and salad that I had prepared. Nancy washed her plate and cutlery and returned to the teak table with her bedtime pill bottle. Instead of taking her medication directly from the pharmacy's Dispill blister pack, she routinely transferred the pills into four plastic bottles for breakfast, lunch, dinner and bedtime. Rarely did she miss a dose; no one could accuse her of being careless (I have defended her on this issue more than once). That evening, her hands were shaking badly. She held the pill bottle sideways and struggled to open the lid, refusing my help. Finally, the lid popped off and two tiny white pills rolled onto the floor. We bent over to pick them up at the same time.

"Let me get them," she said.

Nancy was right about our parents' ancient sofa. The cushions had hardened with age. I spent the night in a series of clockwise turns while she snored lightly on her brand-new Sealy Posturepedic mattress. At the first hint of daylight, I dressed and slipped out for a quick run. The front door was unlocked when I returned twenty minutes later. I kicked off my sneakers and knocked on the bathroom door.

"Want a bagel?"

"I wish I could go for a run."

"Is that a yes or a no?"

"I can't do anything with this bum knee."

Arthritis had struck Nancy much younger than it had our father. The orthopedic specialist warned that a knee replacement was a serious procedure, more complicated than a hip. He had repeatedly postponed Nancy's knee replacement to the point where she would soon need a cane. I dropped a bagel into the toaster. A minute later, the condo was infused with sesame.

"I'll have what you're having," she called out from the bathroom, "with coffee."

The coffee was already on. I spread a thick layer of cream cheese on the bagel halves, sliced a banana, drizzled two bowls of plain yogurt with non-pasteurized honey and carried our breakfast to the balcony on our mother's silver-plated tea tray. Nancy was waiting at the bistro table, brushing her hair. She frowned at the plate I set in front of her.

"I don't eat a big breakfast," she said.

I'd never inquired about Nancy's diet when she was part of the family at L'Abri. Geoff made meals, the apartment volunteers organized cooking nights and Nancy often ate in restaurants.

"A good breakfast regulates blood sugar. Don't forget about your type 2 diabetes."

"Why would I forget? It's my body, remember?"

"Just trying to help."

"Guess I need to buy groceries."

"For sure. What will you buy?"

"Bran flakes, bananas."

"Hmmm. No protein on that list."

"I know more about proper diet than you."

For years Nancy had met with a nutritionist, an outpatient service offered by the Douglas Hospital. She eventually quit, claiming that she knew as much as the dieticians. I had no doubt that was true. Still, her eating habits worried me, especially now that she was living alone. I picked up my coffee and leaned over the balcony railing. I'd been trying hard to stay positive. My patience was wearing thin.

"You must have liked the pasta I made for us last night. You ate it all."

"So?"

I sighed. "So, nothing."

"I need more coffee," said Nancy.

"In a sec. When I finish mine."

"How long will that take?"

"Why don't you serve yourself? I'm not the maid."

"I thought you were here for me."

I turned to face her.

"Seriously?"

"There's not much light in the condo," Nancy said, changing the subject.

None of the apartments and condos we'd visited had been very bright. The size and layout of this one, however, had the others beaten. Did she not remember that? I gave up. Time to go. I carried my coffee and breakfast dishes to the kitchen sink. Nancy followed me inside.

"What am I supposed to do today?" she asked.

I washed and rinsed my mug and plate and placed them on the new drainboard.

"Dunno. Check out the neighbourhood. Have a snack at one of those cafés a few blocks from here."

"The cafés are too far."

"There's one two blocks west on Sherbrooke. Or take a bus. Go to

Atwater. Go downtown. Get out. It'll be good for you."

"You don't need to give me orders. You're not my boss."

"Believe me, the last thing I want is to be your boss."

I refilled her mug and returned the pot to the machine too quickly, leaving a trail of coffee drips on the floor.

"You made a mess!" she cried.

"I'm sure you are capable of cleaning up."

I grabbed my overnight bag and marched out the door. Nancy called from her doorway.

"Thank you for everything, darling sister!"

I wasn't fooled by the fake sweetness in her voice, not for one second. She was blasé and ungrateful even though I'd bent over backwards to make her comfortable. If not me, who else would co-sign the lease, move the furniture, pay the rent and utilities, care about what she ate or didn't eat? Unlike her, I never wanted to be the boss, and I certainly wasn't lording my power over her as she once did to me.

I shivered from a memory when we were six and nine. We had dressed up as "mother and baby" for a costume contest organized by a summer day camp. Nancy's lips were painted red and she wore our mother's floral housedress with large pink buttons. The hem brushed against Nancy's ankles even though our mother had cut off six inches. She glimmered with costume jewellery: a diamond broach pinned to her chest, emeralds dangling from her ears, a string of pearls around her neck.

"How come you're allowed to wear Mom's fancy things?" I asked.

"Because I'm the grown-up."

With great reluctance, I climbed into an old buggy my sister used for her dolls. The faded canopy was torn in several places and the steel frame groaned under my weight.

"I'm too big. It's gonna break!" I cried.

She handed me an old woollen baby blanket that reeked of mothballs. I reminded myself of the red ribbon we might win while my sister tucked the scratchy blanket around my neck and handed me a pacifier that tasted like the rubber on a pencil top. I peered at the streak of blue sky through a tear in the canopy. The buggy groaned down Tettenhall Road. At the end of the block, a wheel caught on the edge of the sidewalk.

"Be careful!" I cried.

Nancy scolded me in a fake adult voice.

"Babies don't talk!"

The day camp was swarming with pirates, witches and monsters. Our costumes felt ordinary. How would we compete with Superman? Nancy whispered commands: stay still, curl up your legs, hold the blanket to your neck. She pushed the buggy across the field towards the picnic table full of counsellors. One of them peered down at me.

"What a lovely baby boy!"

I spat out the pacifier.

"I'm a girl!" I shouted.

The counsellor laughed and my sister's knee pressed into the buggy against the crown of my head, a silent reminder that babies don't talk. He pinned a red ribbon to Nancy's housedress. Her cheeks flushed and her eyes beamed with victory. I propped myself up on an elbow for a better view. My heart sank. Everyone was pinned with a red ribbon. Fingers pointed at me. Kids were laughing. I wrapped the blanket around my bare chest, humiliated and furious, stuck in the buggy. Powerless.

I hurried down Benny with the unpleasant memory and the overnight bag bumping against my thigh. Three blocks later, my pace slowed. The loss of power I'd experienced in the baby buggy was fleeting, like childhood. My sister's loss of control was permanent, an adult reality. The illness kept her captive in an ongoing and pointless struggle for power. The move to the condo had aggravated her—all the things I'd done for her that she could not do for herself. She needed time to calm and adjust to the new situation. Maybe tomorrow she would feel more positive about her home. Maybe she would be more gracious about my support. Maybe we could meet at a cute café on Sherbrooke. Meanwhile, I needed a proper sleep. Our parents' rattan sofa had hurt my back.

The promised home visits from the CLSC clinic kicked in two months after Nancy had moved into the condo; the wait time felt very long. The frail, thirty-year-old CLSC caseworker struggled to understand my sister's loosely associated thoughts. I suggested that Nancy speak in English, but she refused; the caseworker was obviously more comfortable with French. The frequency of the home visits tapered off as the year progressed. The caseworker was often on sick leave—burnout, I assumed. At the end of the second year, we were informed that Nancy was no longer eligible. Her file had been closed. The CLSC didn't see the point in continuing since Nancy had refused to establish "objectives" the caseworker could assist with. "Just as well it's over," said Nancy. She didn't need objectives. She needed contact with people. Thankfully, the hole left by the public health-care system was filled by check-in visits from L'Abri and weekly follow-ups with a dedicated caseworker from Cummings Centre, a well-known Jewish social services agency who, I'd discovered, offered mental health support to Montreal residents, Jewish or not. When Nancy's knee replacement was finally scheduled, I arranged for a private homecare worker named Jessica to keep Nancy company. Jessica quickly became part of the family, a spare sister and a huge support in Nancy's life three days a week.

Despite the strong network that fortified my sister three years into her independent living, I still wrestled with her daily demands and growing resentment. Our lives were more entwined than ever. We bickered constantly. The most recent dispute was where to meet up for coffee. We finally agreed on Le Croissanterie, a known caffeine haven for retirees and mothers with strollers. Not my idea of café ambiance, but the cool draft from the ceiling vent was a welcome refuge on a sweltering July afternoon. I slid into the seat across from my sister. Her face was flushed and damp despite the air conditioning.

"Sorry, I'm a bit late."

She checked her watch.

"I've been here seventy-three minutes."

I leaned forward. "Why do you always insist on arriving so early?"

The empty coffee mug jumped from the weight of her fist landing on the table.

"Some of us are perpetually punctual. Some of us are perpetually late."

"Early isn't being punctual."

She thumped a second time, attracting the attention of three white-haired women at the next table. I leaned towards my sister.

"Calm down. People are watching."

"You calm down."

I turned to the women and mouthed, "Sorry." One smiled back. The other two looked away. Nancy's fingers struggled with the zipper on her handbag.

"You should mention your shaking when you see Dr. Byrne tomorrow. Maybe he can reduce the lithium."

"You're coming with me, right?"

"Yes. I'm coming."

My notes for Dr. Byrne were prepared and sitting on my desk back home. Lithium reduction was not the only item on the list. I needed to talk to him about other things.

She gave up on the zipper and dropped the handbag on the floor.

"What did you whisper to those women at the next table? Are you complaining about me?"

"I was apologizing for the noise."

"Is that all you have to worry about? Noise? That's minor compared to my problems."

"I'm going to the counter for a latte. Want anything?"

Nancy picked up an empty cup.

"Had one already."

"How about something to eat?"

"Done that too."

"I suppose you want to leave soon."

"Probably."

"The plan was to have coffee together."

"If you had arrived on time . . ."

My jaw clenched. "I was only ten fucking minutes late."

"Don't say the f-word."

She pushed away from the table. "I'm buying," she said.

I hesitated. The offer didn't feel friendly.

"Thanks, but—"

"Wait here."

I surrendered to her command even though the coffee I so desperately needed would take a while. Nancy had stopped two tables over and was leaning over a wide-eyed toddler in a stroller. She would likely stop at another table before ordering my latte and offer one of her compliments: "Beautiful dress!" or "You have a lovely complexion!"

"Mommy!" the little boy in the stroller cried out. "She says she has a fake leg!"

My sister loved to show off the scar on her knee, although it was less impressive than the one across her abdomen. The orthopedic surgeon's hesitation to operate had been well-founded. I knew something was wrong in the hospital; she was too groggy, unable to perform the post-op exercises. I suspected a medication mishap like the one following Nancy's pancreatectomy. My concerns were ignored, an invisible health-care worker. Finally, a psychiatrist was summoned and the Clozaril dosage was reduced without delay. Apparently, the medical staff on the surgical ward were unaware that when a patient on Clozaril suddenly stops smoking (i.e., when admitted to hospital), Clozaril levels can elevate to toxic levels. More shocking evidence of our siloed health-care system. The medication mishap, combined with Nancy's refusal to follow the physiotherapy, extended an anticipated three-day hospital stay to four weeks.

Nancy delivered my latte, the cup and saucer teetering in her hand. I thanked her and indulged in a generous gulp. The coffee scalded my tongue and I reached for the water glass.

"Did you hear what I just said?" Nancy asked.

I shook my head.

"I repeat, my television remote isn't working and the window crank in the bedroom is broken."

"Did you ask Jessica for help?"

"She said to ask you."

Helping with the condo didn't bother me. Nor did I mind the administrative duties or advocating for her mental and physical health, the endless medical appointments. The interactions, however, had become back-breaking—the endless phone calls, the problems she needed me to solve, the berating, the complaints, the jealousy, the bitter resentment. Had she ever loved me? Jessica had recently shared her secret trick with me. She let Nancy do whatever Nancy wanted. No power struggle. Easy to do when you aren't family.

"Okay, I'll deal with it."

"When?"

"Later today."

She picked up her handbag from the floor.

"I have to go."

"Okay, bye," I said, fuming.

I moved to a table beside the window, opened my journal and added to my intentions list: *See friends more often.* Five minutes later, someone tapped on the glass. Nancy was waving from the sidewalk with a big grin, like she'd done something clever. She had left the café but was still there, and she had my full attention. Annoying as hell. I downed the rest of my coffee and added *Reduce visits with my sister to once a week* to the list. Nancy was peering through the glass. I packed up my belongings and joined her on the sidewalk.

"You're welcome for the coffee," she said.

"I already thanked you."

"No, you didn't."

"Yes, I did."

"Where are you going?" she asked.

"Home."

"Walking?

"Yup."

"You're lucky to get exercise."

I sighed. "Why don't you walk home too? You live much closer."

"I'm handicapped."

"That's ridiculous. Your knee is perfectly good."

"How do you know what my knee feels like?"

I stepped up to her, inches from her face.

"Remind me why we bothered meeting today?"

"I had time to kill."

"You know, you're right. I have no idea what your knee feels like. *And I really don't give a crap!*"

I turned in the direction of home and hurtled down the block with the hope of distancing myself from the inevitable blast.

"*Go home to your sucker husband!*"

It was the lowest of blows. Something snapped inside me, much deeper than the heart. My soul perhaps. I leaned against a mailbox. The city was spinning around me. She was still within earshot, screaming mean things.

That evening, once my world had calmed, another intention was added to my list: *Avoid saying things that trigger her.* Nancy called ten minutes later.

"Sorry," she said. Her voice sounded soft, genuine.

"Me too."

"The bathroom sink's dripping."

"How much?"

"A little."

"I'll call the plumber in the morning."

"I have no cash to pay him."

"I can do an e-transfer."

"A what?"

"I can pay him through the internet."

"I wouldn't know about that highfalutin arrangement."

"Not highfalutin, just technology. Listen, Nancy, I gotta go. Let's talk tomorrow."

She called back an hour later.

"Did you call the landlord about the window crank?" she asked.

"Shit. I forgot."

"You have other priorities than me."

"I'm tired."

"I guess I'm not important."

Here we go again and again and again.

I made the calls about the television and the window crank and left a message for the plumber; it was the only way to get rid of her for a while. The social worker from the Burgess Pavilion was right: I enabled my sister. Why should I accompany her to Dr. Byrne the next morning? Why subject myself to more verbal abuse? My caring intentions had pulled me into an emotional whirlpool that was threatening my survival. If I didn't break away from the downward spiral soon, I would be sucked into nothing. We would both drown, a tragic end to our sick sisterhood journey. I was fed up with my sister, even more with myself.

But I couldn't step away. What if something happened? She lived alone. I was the point person. Who else would catch her when she fell? I knew damn well I would go with her to the appointment with Dr. Byrne, that I wouldn't be able to get one word in except to mention the shaking from the lithium, that I would have to sit and listen to her remarks. Surely she will mention that she has only been invited twice to the cottage this summer. Afterwards, I will drive her home feeling diminished and small, pulled further than ever into the deep end that she once saved me from. Forever in her debt. Why would my life ever change?

Keith and I had returned from the Rio Grande a narrow five days before Premier Legault's March 14 declaration of a province-wide public health emergency. Infections from Covid-19 were skyrocketing in Quebec. Schools were closed. Flights and trains were cancelled. My writing workshop was switched to Zoom. Nancy's weaving was placed on hold. The city was buzzing from the threat of a lockdown. Earlier that morning, Keith had packed his truck and left for the Eastern Townships with a promise from me to join him in a few hours. I needed to say goodbye to my sister.

Traffic on Sherbrooke was unusually light. Cars lined both sides of Benny, a sign that residents were staying close to home. I parked under the leafless maple across from my sister's front windows (her only windows, she would aptly correct me). The tree had grown several feet higher in the three-and-a-half years she'd been living there. I grabbed the shopping bag and stepped onto the sidewalk. Nancy was wearing a navy-blue windbreaker, a thin layer for pre-spring weather. She walked towards me. I pulled my grey wool beanie over my ears and held up my hand.

"We can't get any closer. Too risky."

"Not much tan," said Nancy.

I touched my cheek, remembering the bamboo raft on the river.

"Is that for me?" she asked and pointed at the shopping bag in my hand.

I lowered the bag to the sidewalk and stepped back. "We shouldn't get too close."

"But we're family."

"Tell that to the virus."

She walked up to the bag and poked at its contents: our mother's book on Expressionism, a box of oil pastels, bar of soap, cotton socks. Her brow furrowed.

"I need help to carry the bag upstairs."

I looked up at her window.

"Can't you handle it by yourself? I'd rather not go inside."

"You haven't been inside for months."

"Not true!" I wondered if it was . . .

"Do you have any masks?" I asked.

"Of course. I bought three boxes yesterday."

My sister had two more boxes than me. I pointed at her face. "You should be wearing one."

"Why bother? You're not. Nobody is."

She picked up the shopping bag. "Wait for me on the bench by the side door."

"I'm not staying. The car's packed up for the Townships and I want to get over the bridge before rush hour."

Her face clouded over. She was shivering a little in her flimsy windbreaker. I stood on the sidewalk, silent, uncertain, my sister studying me.

"You're leaving me stranded?"

"Don't be dramatic," I said. "You live in a city. I'm the one who'll be isolated. You have visits from Jessica and check-in calls with your case-worker. I'm sure Julie will keep in touch."

"You won't be isolated. You have a husband. But don't worry about me. I'm experienced. This is not exactly my first shut-in."

A flotilla of daycare toddlers was fast approaching, possible Covid carriers, every one of them. My sister shifted the bag to her other hand. She would strike up a conversation with the children, bend down close to their runny noses, unconcerned about social distancing, a term not yet adopted in those early days of the pandemic paradigm. She had no trepidation about a mutated coronavirus. She was braver than me. Or maybe she just didn't care.

I stepped off the curb to dodge the daycare bullets and hurried across the street for safety. My feet slowed as I approached the car. Should I have helped with the heavy shopping bag? Should I have stayed a little longer? The guilt-laden questions usually triggered the whirlpool of emotion that nullified shamanic wisdom, social worker advice, journal entries, promises to my family and my own common sense. For once, the pull was easy to resist. It wasn't the global pandemic that had thrown me a lifeline to step away from my sister responsibilities; I had thrown the life-line to myself. Clutching onto the number one ticket, I sped southbound over the Champlain Bridge.

I arrived at the cottage in eighty minutes, record time. Keith, on snowshoes, waved from the field below. The frost on the spruce moun-tains above him twinkled like diamonds in the late afternoon sun. He stomped up the hill to greet me. His goofy smile was visible even at a distance of one hundred feet. Hurry up! I wanted to tell him. I desper-ately needed a hug. Without the whirlpool, I felt strangely empty. But I also felt strangely good.

25

JUNE 2020. I SPED NORTH TOWARDS THE Champlain Bridge. The Montreal skyline came into view and my heart soared. The city shimmered in light, touched by the sun's magic wand: the mountain, the dome of the oratory, the grain elevators, even the rusted freighter in the St. Lawrence Seaway. Covid-19 was ever-present, but the numbers were falling. After a two-month refuge in the Eastern Townships, I was coming home. Chiming bells rang from the car's audio system. The phone call was perfectly timed.

"Are you on the bridge yet?" asked my sister.

I beamed like a delighted child. "Halfway across! I'll be there in ten."

I parked under the maple, now covered in new leaf and jogged across the street, excited for the reunion. At first, Nancy had resented my decision to hide out in the Eastern Townships. She'd accused me of desertion. Once again, I resisted the pull. We both knew I would never abandon her. As spring progressed, the tone of our phone conversations shifted, the tension lifted. She accepted the situation, the physical distance between us. Our calls became friendly, silly even. She would tell me about the people on the sidewalk she met from her second-floor balcony, one of them was a psychotherapist; the pandemic had opened up a new passerby world my sister has cultivated ever since. Her complaints about me, about her caseworker, about Jessica, about everyone, tapered off except for the occasional remark. She teased me about my constant reminders to sanitize and mask. "Paranoia will destroy ya," she warned and then pointed out that I was more likely to catch Covid being the less hygienic sister. (Nancy is still a Novid super-dodger). The groceries I purchased for her online were graciously received, and after years of resistance, my darling sister finally mastered the TV remote and a flip mobile phone. She scheduled her day around *Friends*, *Murder She Wrote*, the six o'clock news and DJ Tyler Barr's radio show when Tyler played her request—Pharrell Williams's song "Happy."

Nancy and I met at the side door of her condo building. We were dressed in short sleeves and sweatpants, our feet in sandals. Her hair, like mine, had grown several inches. I opened my arms and then clasped them around me in a mock hug.

"You look great!" I shouted.

We lowered our masks and grinned at each other. Nancy turned sideways and straightened her top.

"Check this out. My Clozaril belly is already starting to deflate!"

Nancy had articulated a strong desire to quit Clozaril. Her moods had been stable and the obligatory monthly blood tests potentially exposed her to the virus. The long list of side effects had always made me uneasy. Was there a link between this last-resort drug and the stage 0 leukemia in her blood? I had yet to be given a clear answer. Dr. Byrne suggested a gradual withdrawal ending in the fall. Once off Clozaril, he would replace lithium with Tegretol—a bipolar medication without the side effect of shaking. Nancy was thrilled. I shook my head in wonder. Deprescribing! Leave it to my sister to flourish during a pandemic.

"What's in the bag?" she asked.

"Our lunch. Can we picnic somewhere?"

"I know a place," she said. "Follow me.

We followed a path to a community garden at the backside of her building. Only a few of the allotments were tended, like the one with the Japanese lantern we stopped to admire. I bent down to touch a young tomato plant staked to a wooden trellis. The leaves felt soft and fuzzy between my fingers. The new stem already smelled spicy and sweet. Nancy had recently applied for an allotment. She was thrilled with the idea of planting her own vegetables and pleased that Jessica and Julie had offered to help. We settled on opposite sides of a nearby bench, sister bookends. I pulled out two tuna sandwiches wrapped in tinfoil. A few slices from a homegrown tomato would have gone well.

"Delicious!" Nancy cried. "Thank you!"

"But you haven't taken a first bite!"

"I can tell."

I kicked off my sandals and wiggled my toes. Nancy did the same. The picnic confirmed what I had sensed from our phone conversations. The initial reduction in Clozaril had injected her with a positive energy. Was this the beginning of a new era?

"L'Atelier opens up in a few weeks," Nancy said, her mouth full of tuna.

"Do you want to go?"

She nodded with enthusiasm.

"I've been going to L'Atelier longer than anywhere else. Can't quit now!"

Drenched in sunlight, we lounged on the bench in the community garden and chatted about what vegetables and flowers Nancy would plant. For two magical hours, mental illness and the pandemic did not exist. We parted with smiles. My sister and I had an entire season of picnics ahead of us.

The summer lived up to expectations. Under Nancy's watchful eye, with help from Jessica and Julie, the small allotment in the community garden flourished, especially the cucumbers and cherry tomatoes. Every few weeks, the Clozaril dosage was reduced a little more. It was a cloudy October afternoon when we pulled out the trellis and raked the earth smooth. Nancy and I didn't linger. She was tired. Without the sedating Clozaril in her bloodstream, she was having trouble sleeping.

November 1: daylight savings came to an end. I looked forward to an extra hour of sleep, one of the few perks of November. Instead, chiming bells woke me.

"Kinda early to call, no?" I mumbled.

"I didn't sleep last night." My sister's voice sounded rough.

I threw off the blanket and rubbed my eyes.

"Do you have a fever or a cough?"

"It's not Covid. I just couldn't sleep."

"You probably slept more than you thought."

"I slept an hour at most."

I sat up.

The haunting memory of nighthawks and my sister's insomnia came rushing back. I shook off the past. Three weeks off Clozaril, she was lucid and stable. Nothing to worry about, she would have to learn how to sleep without medication, just like our father did. Welcome to the real world. This was a one-off, just a lousy sleep.

"You'll catch up tonight," I said, stretching my legs.

But she didn't catch up. The insomnia persisted all week and into the one following. I reached out to Dr. Byrne, who prescribed clonazepam, which Nancy described as tiny blue pills that did nothing. Another blue pill was added with no results. They were useless, she said. More time passed. Instead of succumbing to fatigue, she became infused with confidence, not her usual rebellion, but a fierce self-reliance that reminded me of the child sister who pushed me around in the baby buggy.

"I don't need anyone's help," she told me. "I'm taking charge of my life!"

She asked me to cease communications with Dr. Byrne, cancel her online groceries and stop asking how many hours she slept. I was happy to comply. Without my sister figuring front and centre, I was keen to redirect my energy towards new projects, although I felt a little lost as to what they might be.

I continued to watch from the sidelines in awe of her high energy in the face of prolonged sleep deprivation. The mania caused by the dopamine rush from Clozaril withdrawal was more controlled than the extreme rollercoaster ride without lithium. Nancy transferred her prescriptions to a more efficient pharmacy, organized a meeting at the bank to discuss her monthly service fees, kept track of distances walked and stocked her refrigerator with supplies. She was fuelled with confidence to take back power, to give the imposter "sick" sister a swift kick in the ass. "Go, girl, go!" I shouted. My sister didn't hear. She was travelling at the speed of a shooting star, barrelling further and further from my supporting arms that had defined us for so long. I stood at a distance, a bittersweet sadness rising in my heart from the inevitable crash. In the meantime, she deserved to be fully alive.

Nancy called mid-afternoon on winter solstice. We hadn't spoken in days, although I'd learned from the pharmacist that Dr. Byrne had prescribed Haldol to calm her. She was around the corner in Lower Westmount. Was I available? I invited her to our basement, to the other side of a plastic wall we'd constructed from PVC sheeting for the holidays. Nancy was not impressed with our Covid barrier. She described the plastic wall as illegal, against the new restrictions that banned indoor gatherings. Let's meet at Prince Albert Square instead, she said. I pleaded with her to come to the basement. It was freezing outside. I would make tea. She would have access to her own bathroom.

"Meet me at the square," she said.

I zipped up my woollen coat and pulled on a pair of cotton gloves. My heavy winter gear was still packed away with the naive hope that cold weather would hold off until January. At the end of the block, the wind picked up. I flipped up my hood and hurried towards Sherbrooke, thankful for the warmth of the surgical mask. Nancy was alone in the square, brushing her hair at a picnic table that wouldn't be used until spring. Her mitts, hat, mask and shopping bags were beside her on the bench.

"Aren't you cold?" I asked, shifting my feet.

She squinted at me. Her eyes were encircled by shadow.

"Sit down. We can pretend it's one of our picnics."

I adjusted my mask and remained standing.

"Are you nuts? It's too cold to sit. Let's walk!"

"Let me finish my water."

She pulled out a thirty-six-ounce plastic bottle from under the bench and unscrewed the cap. The bottle was heavy, awkward to hold, especially with shaking hands. Water dribbled down the sides of her mouth. I shifted my feet while she drank, feeling the dampness from the pavement through the thin leather soles of my boots. I didn't remind Nancy about her low sodium count, that she shouldn't guzzle down so much water. Finally, she replaced her mask and stood. We crossed to the north side of Sherbrooke and began the steep ascent up the hill. Her banter was constant, the thread impossible to follow. We turned left into Prince Albert Park across from the former house of my childhood friend, Beth. My sister stopped at the first bench. I could no longer feel my toes.

"Can we please keep walking?" I asked, forcing myself to be polite.

She remained seated with complete disregard for my reasonable request. I recognized the familiar ploy for power and resisted its pull. I could leave anytime, walk back down the hill. Turning to face Beth's house, I tried to recapture the warm sunny days, baseball, touch tag, smoking a joint in the playground tunnel. All I could remember were the calls from my parents, the quiet anger I'd felt at being ordered home to help with my sister. The parental voices had died long before their physical shells, as far back as their move to Germany. Their eldest daughter's needs, however, lived on. My vision suddenly blurred. Between dark memories and fogged-up glasses from the mask, I couldn't see a damn thing.

"It's too fucking cold standing here. I'm going home."

I'd taken two steps away from the bench when Nancy began to hurl insults. Her accusations bounced off my skin, falling dead on the cold ground, nothing feeding them. She left the bench with her two shopping bags and steamed in the opposite direction as much as her crooked walk would allow. She turned up the next street and disappeared, leaving me with an old lump in my throat. I chugged up the hill parallel to her route, one block between us. The icy climb was treacherous, especially where the slope steepened. My useless boots slipped three times. I forged on, determined to catch up with her on the next street.

She didn't notice me watching from above. I removed my mask to catch my breath and defog. Her pace slowed. She paused in front of a semi-detached red brick house that looked a lot like our former family home—trimmed conifer on a postage-stamp lawn, side verandah, the wood painted grey, bay windows on the first and second floors. I wondered if she was feeling the same confused nostalgia.

I replaced my mask as she approached. The cotton was soggy from my breath, no longer an effective barrier. She was neither surprised nor pleased to see me. The indifference in her eyes reminded me of our father when I ran out from behind a tree and ambushed him during his solo evening walks, my failed efforts to cheer him up.

"You said you would walk with me." Her voice was icicle-sharp.

"Sitting on benches doesn't qualify as walking. Look at me. I'm freezing!"

"Then go home."

I raised my hand in a salute.

"I think I will."

My gesture might have looked sarcastic, but it was genuine. I was happy to obey. I crossed the street and descended the hill at a fast clip. Nancy miraculously kept pace on the opposite sidewalk, yelling at me between the passing cars until we reached the intersection. I imagined the comfort from the hot tea I would sip in my favourite spot by the dining room window, the glass of wine a couple of hours later. The red light at the intersection glowed under the darkening four o'clock sky. Streetlights came on. I turned and our eyes met. She lowered her mask and smiled. My home was three blocks away. Hers was twenty. Rejecting her friendly overture felt wrong, especially this close to the holidays on the longest night of the year.

I was halfway across the street when her face shifted. The smile had been a ploy. My feet kept moving forward regardless. They stepped onto the curb where she was standing. Her coat was zipped higher now, her toque pulled down. Her scarf was tied in a clumsy knot, the kind a child would make. She stood perfectly still, unaffected by the cold. She had thick skin, the skin of an elephant. I crossed my arms and squeezed them tight to my chest.

"I can't do this anymore. I'm done." My voice cracked like an adolescent.

"Me too, I'm done."

She had rushed her words as if wanting to get there first.

I followed the pedestrians in a diagonal flow across the intersection and took shelter under the awning belonging to L'Occitane en Provence boutique. Their window was decorated with holiday gift baskets lit by a string of delicate white lights. SEULEMENT TROIS CLIENTS À LA FOIS— ONLY THREE CLIENTS AT A TIME was handwritten on a paper taped to the glass, a sign of pandemic times. A customer stepped out of the shop, bringing with her a strong scent of rose and lavender. The perfume neutralized within seconds in the frozen air. Nancy was still on the diagonally opposite corner. She was peering into the empty McDonald's, another casualty of Covid-19. McDonald's was one of her regular stops; she blended into their eclectic patronage. I was not a fan of burgers and fries, but I shared my sister's dislike of the plugged-in clientele at Starbucks. We had that much in common. She cupped her hands and peered through the dark glass as if someone would notice her and unlock the door, offer her a hot beverage to go. I knew my sister's haunts. She would have no trouble finding refuge from the cold on her journey home. A clerk in the Pharmaprix would let her use the employee bathroom. The manager of the takeout pizza restaurant would pour her a glass of water. The cashier at the pet shop would let her use the phone. To call me. She knew how to take care of herself, how to turn the mental illness into an advantage when needed—pandemic or no pandemic.

She bent over her shopping bags with no obvious purpose than to reshuffle the contents. A young man stopped to pick up something she had dropped on the sidewalk. I heard their conversation in my mind. She was explaining how her little sister had gone home to her warm house and husband. My real sister would never have shared personal information, especially with a stranger. The imposter sister hid nothing.

She pushed away from the McDonald's window and removed her

mask and toque, still unaware of my presence. The beam from the streetlamp caught her pale round face. I forgot about the cold, transfixed by the shimmering long hair that looked strawberry blond under the artificial light. I searched for other signs of my real sister, the one who had left at an age when we might have started to become friends, someone to turn to when I'd had my first period, when I felt ugly, when none of the boys I liked had liked me back, when our parents were mean. I often turned the scribbled pages of my teenage diaries looking for references to the imposter sister who had replaced the real one. I never found any. I wanted my real sister back. Why would I care about an imposter?

Nancy straightened, alone in the spotlight. Was it the burning energy of the mania that allowed me to suddenly see her so clearly, not through the distorted lens of illness? Or was it the magic of winter solstice, when the veil between the material and spiritual worlds is at its thinnest? Her slightly crooked posture was imperceptible from where I stood. I imagined the contents of her shopping bags, items organized, everything in order like she kept her home. The scent of soap lingered on her skin from a recent shower. Her hair smelled of lemons. Her hands were rough from scrubbing the bathroom and her kitchen sink. She was diligent and hardworking but also craved human interaction particularly with strangers who didn't know her history. The older sister: responsible, conscientious to a fault. The boss. Annoying at times, nurturing at others. The illness had not succeeded in stealing these qualities. Nancy would not stand for that. We'd been raised in the same strict household, received the same kind of parental love and shared half the same DNA, we were more alike than either of us cared to admit. She knew me like no other, a best friend. This was no imposter. She was the real sister.

Enthused by the realization, I stepped off the curb to tell her, but she pirouetted in an awkward manner and headed west, away from me. Just as well, it was something she probably already knew. She's always been the smarter one.

Nancy turned up Christmas morning. We sat at the tables I had arranged on either side of the plastic wall. She slipped an envelope under the plastic sheeting. There were three holiday cards inside, each one smaller than the one before, like Russian dolls. She asked me to read the greetings out loud. The plastic muffled her voice.

"This isn't much fun," she said.

"Wait, I have something for you," I replied. "Hold on."

I cranked the volume on my phone and pressed play for the "Happy" song. Recognizing the first few beats, she jumped to standing and raised her arms above her head. I followed her lead. We turned in circles, waving our arms and kicking our feet. The plastic wall melted away as we lifted from the ground. We were floating on air, pulled higher and higher. "My level's too high to bring me down." Our sister dance.

She left after the song ended, no mention of where she was headed. Our call that evening was brief. Then the calls stopped altogether. A week later she instructed the driver of the ambulance she'd summoned to take her to Jewish General Hospital. Someone had told her they have an excellent psychiatry department. She refused to rise from the stretcher at emergency, a ploy to avoid the waiting room and to hasten triage. The paramedics caught onto her and walked away muttering. In spite of her efforts, she was transferred to emergency at the Douglas the next morning. Nancy had arranged her own private lockdown.

26

I MISSED THE CHIMING BELLS and my sister's voice, the way we called each other darling. I even missed our fights. Five days and she still hadn't called; the overcrowded emergency room more than satisfied her need to talk. My thoughts drifted back to her throughout the day, while preparing a meal, walking with a friend, sitting at my desk. In the middle of the night, I woke up in a panic that she had left forever. I couldn't imagine life without her.

The hospital staff was difficult to reach, squeezed between slashed budgets and patient overload. An attendant finally answered the phone; her immigrant French was challenging to follow, her English even worse. The undertones of her gravelly voice were, however, crystal clear—lousy pay, double shifts, stressful work conditions. I hung up, sympathetic and no further informed of my sister's condition. The next morning I brought Nancy's flip phone and charger to the hospital along with a few toiletries. Every item was labelled with her name. The stone-faced security guard checked my bag. He asked me to remove my coat and lift my arms. I assumed there had been an incident, a visitor carrying a sharp object. But lift my arms? Did he think I was aiding and abetting? The social worker from Burgess who had accused me of enabling would laugh at that.

Emergency was not a place to heal; it was a holding cell until a bed became available elsewhere. Living in a chaotic environment without treatment, Nancy's agitation escalated even higher. On day five she was transferred to *soins intensifs* (intensive care), a smaller emergency unit with larger problems. The attendant unlocked the door so I could visit in Nancy's room, an exception to their rule given the enraged 250 pound male patient roaming the hall. The staff condoned his screaming and banging rather than drag him into the side room—an improvement from Perry 2C days. I sat on the edge of the narrow mattress, wincing every time his fist met the wall. My sister was too agitated to care, oblivious to the nightmarish surroundings, including her claustrophobic room with faded graffiti on the yellowed walls, messages written with illicit pens belonging to former inmates. *I pooped in my pants last week and my mother shamed me for it . . . I love you Marge. I'm sorry and I actually like your glasses. You're very pretty.* The brief visit, like the others, ended with my expulsion. "LEAVE!" I was happy to obey her demand.

On the tenth day, Nancy was transferred to a pavilion called Porteous, an Anglo-Norman French name meaning "something carried out of doors." My sister wouldn't be outdoors for a while. The attending psychiatrist reached out to me almost immediately. "I want to learn more about your sister," he said over the phone. I beamed inside, no longer an invisible health-care partner. He was soft-spoken and listened attentively while I shared the history, shocked to learn that the number in her file referring to a thirteen-year hospital stay was not a typo.

"Would it be okay if I prescribed Clozaril?" he asked Nancy during our in-person meeting the following week. I sat quietly without an agenda or a list. Nancy was in charge of her own care.

She hesitated.

"What about my low sodium levels? I'm thirsty all the time and they won't let me drink water!"

She was trying her best to obfuscate even though the sodium problem was real. Her mouth sounded parched, the way her tongue clicked when she spoke. A week later, Nancy would be rushed by ambulance to the Verdun Hospital for a forty-eight-hour sodium drip; it was a shame that the procedure could not be performed in a psychiatric institution. The transfer between hospitals would set her mental health recovery back a week, maybe more.

"Yes, your sodium levels are low. We suspect this is caused by Tegretol. We're monitoring you closely. Is it okay if we start you on Clozaril?"

"I'm having problems with my roommate. She stole my T-shirt. She denies it, but I know she did."

"She's not easy, your roommate. Let me speak to the staff. Thank you for letting me know." The doctor then added, "I suggest we start with

217

twenty-five milligrams and see how that goes. Is that okay with you?"

She shrugged. Her efforts to avoid the question had failed.

"Sure."

Back on Clozaril was a backwards move. "It's a low dose," I whispered, grabbing her hand. She shooed me away. My sympathy wasn't helpful.

The starting dose was increased gradually over the next eight weeks. Nancy complained of a Clozaril belly and oversedation. Her speech slowed and her agitation waned. She was still prone to outbursts, but they were triggered by outside circumstances including an unwarranted attack by the difficult roommate who had since been moved.

"How are you feeling, Nancy?" the psychiatrist asked during our second in-person meeting.

She placed her hands, palms down, on the conference table and leaned towards him.

"Much better as you can see. When may I leave?"

"If all goes well, you should be ready for discharge early next week, after the Easter long weekend. But first, I'd like to arrange a supervised day pass. We can see how that goes."

My stomach tightened. A day pass?

"How many hours?" I asked.

"How about one o'clock to seven? Are you available?"

Six hours was a hell of a long visit. We usually lasted only two. I pictured myself enduring the beratement and criticism, Saint Susan carrying the cross on her back. It was an ancient story, one appropriate for Easter weekend. I thought of asking Keith and the kids for help. They could change their weekend plans. Then I came to my senses; this was my responsibility, not theirs.

"I could pick Nancy up tomorrow, on Good Friday . . ."

"Perfect! I'll arrange the paperwork."

Nancy remained silent. Was she thinking what I was thinking? What the hell would we do for six hours?

"Maybe we could hang out at my place?" I suggested as she walked me to the door.

"Not your place," she muttered.

Understandable. Too many negative associations, all those sister fights.

"How about your place then?"

She shook her head. We parted without a plan.

A little after one o'clock on Good Friday, I climbed the stairs to the second floor of the Porteous Pavilion and pressed on the buzzer. Within seconds, Nancy's face popped up on the other side of the glass window. I smiled. My ever-ready sister on the lookout. I didn't need reinforcement from my partner or my children. I had her. The excitement in her voice penetrated the thick steel of the locked door.

"She's here! My sister is here!"

The lock clicked open and the handle turned. She scooted out like a cat escaping, her blond hair tied in a high ponytail. She was wearing familiar black leggings with her grey hoodie and lace-up boots I'd never seen before. The three-inch heels were a striking deviation from her usual sneakers. She mentioned where the boots came from, a store I'd never heard of.

"Say that again?" I asked. "What boutique?"

"Soins Intensifs," she repeated slowly. "Intensive care."

We paused to laugh, then descended the staircase at a relaxed pace, five hours and fifty minutes remaining in the day pass. I pulled open the main door.

"It's chilly out. You'll need a coat. I have one for you in the car."

She waved a hand in the air, a dismissal.

"Don't tell me what I need, thank you very much."

"Suit yourself."

She took the lead, tottering across the parking lot in her second-hand heels, refusing my assistance to climb into the car. We cruised at a leisurely speed through the hospital grounds and turned right onto boulevard Champlain without an itinerary. I merged onto the expressway while Nancy stared out the window at the passing urban landscape with the curiosity of someone who hadn't seen their homeland in a while. I considered the possibility that we could drive around all afternoon.

"Should I get off at Atwater?" I asked. "We could check out Atwater Market."

"Sure."

Nancy pointed at a sign. "Turn right here," she said. "For Atwater."

"Not a good idea. That'll take us onto the Champlain Bridge."

"You're wrong. I've taken a hundred taxis this way."

I kept silent, leaving her the last word but ignoring her instructions. I took the second right turn, praying that the market would be open on Good Friday.

"Let's go to the car wash instead," she said, pointing at the gas station on the corner of Atwater and Notre Dame.

"Are you serious?"

"When did you last wash this car? It looks pretty dirty!"

I'd forgotten how, months earlier, the line-up for the automated car wash on Notre Dame had been too long and neither one of us had the patience to wait.

"Good idea!" I pulled into the gas station, filled up the tank and joined the queue. Six cars were ahead of us.

"Are you sure you want to spend your day pass doing this?"

"I'm sure."

Ten minutes later, the line had advanced by only one car length. Two vehicles had pulled in behind us, too late for a change of mind. I looked over at Nancy. She seemed content. Clozaril had vanquished the mania. I patted her leg, an affectionate tap.

She pulled away. "Stop touching me like that. It's patronizing."

"Should I play some music?"

My suggestion was sanctioned by a nod. I clicked on a Bob Marley playlist, a favourite of mine.

"Don't like that. Play something else."

"Tell me what you want to hear."

"Not that!"

Three more playlists were rejected until we agreed on the "Happy" song. She crossed her arms and listened, a blank expression on her face. I wondered if there was a fire burning inside. If there was, I hadn't stoked it. I pulled ahead another car length and played her song a second time. Finally, our turn arrived. I lowered the window to punch in the code on my gasoline receipt.

"You're so smart with these things," she said, her voice edged with resentment.

The garage door lifted, then closed behind us when we had advanced far enough. Seconds later, we were enveloped in a kaleidoscope of soapy foam. "Look at those crazy colours!" I cried. Nancy looked straight ahead, nonplussed. Had the medication dampened her senses? High-pressure jets circled the car. I counted six slow rotations, which explained the line-up of cars outside; the rinse cycle was ridiculously long. I glanced at the clock, certain that we'd been washed enough. Trapped in a small space, an old sense of unease returned. My eyes fixed on the red light, waiting for the green signal. I was more than ready to leave. Was this how Nancy felt about the hospital?

"I hope the equipment isn't malfunctioning. This is taking forever," I said quietly, aware of the thumping in my chest.

She squeezed my shoulder. "Think of your shiny clean car."

I relaxed a little, her reassuring hand resting on my shoulder. Finally, the garage door lifted and my heart calmed. We advanced through the blast of hot air onto the street, three-and-a-half hours remaining in the day pass.

"Where to now, Nance?" I asked, blinking in the daylight.

"I have a craving for dumplings, that place near your house."

We parked a convenient two blocks from MeiWei Dumpling on Sherbrooke ouest. Stepping onto the sidewalk, I zipped up my jacket, knowing better not to mention the extra coat lying on the back seat. Nancy's icy hand slipped inside my jacket pocket. We walked like that, huddled together, our arms linked, her fingers wrapped around mine hidden from public view, slowed by the crooked walk that had deteriorated in the hospital. People smiled as they passed. I wondered what they saw. Two sisters holding each other up? We lingered over the plate of dumplings at MeiWei, tasting the various sauces and studying their ingredients. Time passed, two hours remaining.

"Where to next?" I asked.

She grinned, a little girl smile. "I want a chocolate Easter bunny. We could pick one up at Pharmaprix."

I made a face. "We can do better than the pharmacy. Let's try the new bakery. It's only a block away."

She looked skeptical, but her hand slipped back into my pocket. We continued along Sherbrooke, pausing for brief conversations with a dog, a baby, a parent. The new bakery was located on the same intersection where I had discovered my real sister on winter solstice. Four months later, the stars had aligned once again; the bakery offered a cornucopia of artisanal holiday chocolate. Nancy purchased a ten-inch Easter bunny and two lattes, which I carried to a table by the window. In the booth next to us a father sat across from his young teenage daughter. The girl's pretty dark eyes were vacant and glazed. She stared at a blank spot on the wall above her father's head while he engaged in a one-way discussion. Nancy didn't notice or she didn't let on. We sipped our coffees and chewed on pieces of chocolate bunny crafted with the perfect amount of sweetness. I checked my phone, only thirty minutes remaining.

"Time to leave," Nancy said.

We were both quiet on the drive back to the hospital, a little worn out and much relieved. The day pass had been a success. I followed Nancy up the stairs to the steel door.

"Take it easy," she said and squeezed my shoulder like she had done in the car wash. "You worry too much."

I was tempted to tell her about the therapist I was seeing, the one she had rejected.

"That was a Good Friday," I said instead.

She smiled at my silly joke, hugged me and then she was gone.

Turning in the opposite direction from the parking lot, I meandered down the hospital road, crossed boulevard LaSalle and reached the river footpath that I'd never taken. I paused a few feet from the water's edge. Rapids danced with the spring thaw. Chunks of ice still hugged the shoreline. It was dusk, the time of day that dipped my mood once upon a time. I didn't know what the future held, how her body would react to the last-resort Clozaril. She was resilient, possibly more resilient than me. My sister would always be the stronger swimmer. I continued along the shoreline with my hand pushed deep in my coat pocket feeling Nancy's fingers holding mine.

ACKNOWLEDGMENTS

Mad Sisters is a project I resisted for years; many of the scenes were painful to revisit. Thank you, Nancy, big sister, for the lessons learned, hard and soft, and for continuing to walk the world with me. To my brave and spirited children, Sarah and Willy, thank you for reminding me that anything is possible, including this book. For my parents, wherever you are, I hold deep appreciation for your suffering and hard work. I miss you. Thank you, precious friends/soul family, for anchoring me with love. Special thanks to my publisher at Ronsdale Press, Wendy Atkinson, for your compassionate support of a mental health narrative that challenges our imperfect social systems and raises awareness about family caregivers. I am indebted to my highly skilled editors, Robyn So and Jennifer Hale. Authors Susan Doherty and Claire Holden Rothman, thank you for encouraging me to write. I'm grateful for caregiver support from AMI-Quebec and Mad in America. A shout-out to Jaime Koss and the writer's group in Sámara, Costa Rica; it's your fault that I quit my day job! Finally, dear partner Keith, my heartfelt appreciation for your unfaltering support, attentive reading, brilliant suggestions and kind tolerance of my erratic writing schedule.

ABOUT THE AUTHOR

Inspired by the *pura vida* while living in Costa Rica, Susan Grundy veered from her 30-year career in marketing to write stories about the weight of emotional distress and how to step into an easier way of being. After her short fiction appeared in the *Danforth Review* and *Montréal Writes*, Susan dove into *Mad Sisters*, a highly personal account of her caregiving journey for an older sister diagnosed with schizophrenia at the age of thirteen. She has completed a second novel (fiction) about an architect who breaks free from a painful ancestral cycle in her female lineage. The present-day story is interlaced with historical vignettes of Susan's farmer ancestors who fled religious persecution in seventeenth-century Europe and eventually found sanctuary near Black Creek in North York, Toronto. When not at her desk, Susan can be found walking in nature towards a café. She divides her time between Montreal and London.